In praise of integrated medicine and Dr

"I am delighted that Dr Mosaraf Ali has written his first book on integral health and medicine. This publication will enable a much wider audience to benefit from his knowledge, wisdom and experience."
HRH The Duchess of Gloucester

"Dr Ali has saved me from pain and from painkillers and their side effects." **Eve Arnold**

"I've been looked after by Dr Ali for eight years and throughout that time I've felt younger every day." **Earl of Dartmouth**

"This is a man...who turned my life around from being overweight, suffering panic attacks to a person full if vim and vigour – way beneath my actual years." **Johnny Gold**

"Dr Ali has the rare talent to associate the best of natural traditional homoeopathic medicine with modern allopathic medicine."
Isabel Goldsmith

"If you are in business these days you are going to be under continuous, extreme stress – and the global economy won't slow down and make life easier for you. But talking to Dr Ali will! Following the simple advice he gave me the first time I met him changed the whole of my life." **Mike Harris**

"Having been bent double getting off a plane in Hong Kong with a slipped disk, I was very sceptical when I arrived at Dr Ali's clinic. I walked out in total amazement half an hour later."
Stephen Marks

"Dr Ali is the Eighth Wonder of the World personified."
Tara Palmer-Tomkinson

"If Hippocrates had needed a doctor he would have sent for this man."
Selina Scott

"Dr Ali's greatest integration are his eyes and hands which often laser through the unhealthy parts of us." **David Tang**

The Integrated Health Bible
The revolutionary healing programme for optimum wellbeing and vitality

Dr Mosaraf Ali

with
Ken Bridgewater

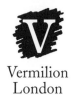

Vermilion
London

3 5 7 9 10 8 6 4

Text © Dr Mosaraf Ali 2001

Dr Mosaraf Ali has asserted his right to be identified as the author of this work under the Copyright, Designs and Patent Act 1988.

First published in 2001 by Vermilion
an imprint of Ebury Press
Random House, 20 Vauxhall Bridge Road, London SW1V 2SA

Random House Australia (Pty) Limited
20 Alfred Street, Milsons Point, Sydney, New South Wales 2061, Australia

Random House New Zealand Limited
18 Poland Road, Glenfield, Auckland 10, New Zealand

Random House South Africa (Pty) Limited
Endulini, 5A Jubilee Road, Parktown 2193, South Africa

The Random House Group Limited Reg. No. 954009

A CIP catalogue record for this book is available from the British Library.

ISBN 0 09 185626 4

Printed and bound in Great Britain by Butler and Tanner Ltd, Frome, Somerset

Papers used by Vermilion are natural, recyclable products made from wood grown in sustainable forests.

To all those who helped me to reach where I am today

CONTENTS

ACKNOWLEDGEMENTS

I am grateful to Jonathan Newhouse at Condé Nast for introducing me to Ed Victor, my agent, who worked hard to convince Random House that my work merited a book.

I am particularly grateful to Ken Bridgewater who went through hours of recordings and pages of scribbled writings, that I had done mostly at night with a tired body and electrified mind. Thanks to his efforts the book was written within four months.

I also wish to express my thanks to Amelia Thorpe and her entire team at Random House for making the book possible.

I am also grateful to those friends who sent me quotes to help promote this book and who supported my ideas.

Finally, I am grateful to HRH the Prince of Wales for writing a Foreword. I hope this will launch me once again into another phase of my work.

INTRODUCTION

My maternal grandfather, Dr Abdul Hameed, was a conventional doctor who specialised in homeopathy and integrated the two systems of medicine. My early memories go back to those times when I used to watch him examine patients – looking at their tongue and eyes, feeling their pulse – before prescribing medicines. He used often to open up anatomical books and teach me about muscles, bones, heart and various organs. My favourite game as a toddler was to play a doctor, imitating my grandfather.

It was then my interest in folk medicine grew. In our own village there was no doctor so people managed their ailments and emergency medical situations with folk or traditional medicine. A man bitten by a venomous cobra, a child unconscious after drowning, a mentally-ill woman, a cholera epidemic, a fracture and joint dislocation – were all treated or managed by traditional medicine right before my eyes. I myself was treated with leeches on my abdomen and a tree bark concoction prepared in goat's milk, for a chronic diarrhoea which even my grandfather could not treat.

In Calcutta, where I attended early school, I would go every Sunday with the domestic servants to the Chowringhee grounds near the Monument. Thousands of people and traders would gather there, as if it were a fair. Afghan herbalists sold their traditional herbs and minerals; teeth were extracted with primitive tools; ears were cleaned with aromatic oils; chronic ailments were treated with copper capsules or amulets containing Quranic verses; arthritis and swelling in the feet treated with molten fat of monitor lizards; hot needles were pierced in points on the skin to eliminate pain in the limbs; and spiritual healing was done by a bearded man in long flowing robes. I saw yogis with their heads buried in the soil and feet upright in the air; sadhus or priests walking on hot charcoal for spiritual purification or lying on a bed of barbed wire or thorns while covered in white ash.

Early in the morning hundreds of Calcuttan Hindu traders would go to the banks of the Hooghly (a tributary of the Ganges) to have a dip in the holy waters. First their bodies would be greased with mustard oil while skinny men would slide up and down their bodies massaging them with their knees and ankles. Fresh mud would then be rubbed all over them before finally they went for their dip in the river. The rich silt of the Ganges contains many minerals and useful algae.

I went to a Christian Brothers' boarding school in Asansol, some 200 km from Calcutta. It was run by Irish and Australian Brothers who were strict but very committed to instilling the correct values in a boy. I was always first in my class and received a scholarship amounting to highly subsidised school fees. My dream to become a doctor was always strong. During the holidays I would spend hours in the United States Information Service Library in Calcutta reading books in psychology, physiology and anatomy. Rather a strange occupation for a 12-year-old!

I met Mother Teresa who, in those days, ran a leprosy centre near the school grounds. On most Sundays when she came down from Calcutta, I helped her Sisters of Charity pack powdered US aid milk for the leprosy sufferers. The mutilated hands and feet were quite shocking to look at and the sisters dressed them with sulfonamide once a week.

Such was the attention I received from the Brothers that biology was introduced in school especially for me as this was an essential subject for a future course in medicine. As part of my school project, I caught some 20 frogs at night, forced a measured amount of alcohol on them and studied their weight loss, breathing rate, oxygen consumption, etc, over 36 hours, staying awake to make recordings every four hours. I put the results into graphs and sent the project to a national science-talent search organisation to win a scholarship. But my first experience with medical practice was when, after my school-leaving exams, I joined a Jesuit paramedic priest and worked in a remote tribal area of Bihar dressing wounds and distributing medicines in different villages.

I joined the University of Delhi for a premedical course, living with my cousin and brother-in-law who was a Congress Member of Parliament. Later I joined a medical college in Delhi but unfortunately my father, who had been a great inspiration to me in my dream to become a doctor, then died. I therefore applied – along with tens of thousands of applicants – for a government scholarship to study medicine in Moscow. Fortunately, I was one of the two selected in the process.

The Dean of the Faculty of Medicine, Professor Yuri Romashoff, was an eminent Soviet cardiac surgeon and yet he was deeply interested in fasting therapy, iridology, tongue diagnosis and yoga. He therefore encouraged students to study these subjects. Although I was deeply interested in them, I was determined to be a good general physician first. In my first year I joined a research scholar to study the early stages of development of rheumatism in mice. Later I became the President of the Students' Scientific Council, encouraging students to participate in research and present papers at conferences. I was the best student of the faculty for four consecutive years.

In my final year of study, Mr Inder Gujral, the then Indian Ambassador in Moscow who later became the Prime Minister of India, asked me to take a visiting Sikh spiritual leader around Moscow. On his final day, this gentleman asked me what I intended to do after completion of my MD studies. I spoke of neurosurgery and he said I should study naturopathy and Ayurveda. Later he sent some books on these subjects which I found 'unscientific' and boring. However Mr Gujral insisted that I follow his advice as he was Maharaj Charan Singh, the spiritual head of Radhasoami group with several million followers.

Using his influence on the Soviet Minister of health, Mr Petrovski, Mr Gujral found me a course in acupuncture. I thus became the first foreigner to be admitted to a postgraduate course at the Central Institute of Advanced Medical Studies where classified subjects like cosmic medicine, parapsychology, experimental medicine, etc, were studied. My supervisor was Inna Petrovna Chkalova, the daughter-in-law of the legendary Soviet test pilot Valerie Chkalov (who flew from Leningrad to Vancouver nonstop over the Arctic in the 1950s and under the Nevsky Bridge in a jet fighter). Inna Petrovna taught me iridology, tongue diagnosis, pulse diagnosis and sent me numerous patients on whom I could practise my skills and gather experience. I had my own full clinic.

During my postgraduate studies I also met Professor Yuri Nikolaev, the father of the Soviet school of fasting therapy and naturopathy. Prof Nikolaev opened up my mind and helped me to believe in the natural healing power in every person.

I concluded my thesis on the treatment of peptic ulcers with acupuncture based on studies carried out on 105 patients and returned to India in 1982. There I joined a hospital in Delhi and a family friend Pranab Mukherjee in whose house I lived, helped me to open a private clinic of my own. He was then a senior minister in Mrs Indira Gandhi's government holding both the Finance and Commerce portfolios. It was during that period I spent most of my spare time with eminent vaidyas (physicians of Ayurveda) and hakims (physicians of Unani). Amongst them was Hakim Abdul Hameed, the last of the masters of Unani, who ran the Hamdard Foundation and later the Hamdard University. It was with utmost devotion I watched him diagnose complicated medical conditions with pulse studies. In later years he gave me a collection of books and said I should one day write about Unani medicine. I am very grateful to him in many ways.

My association with His Holiness Satguru Jagjit Singh, the spiritual head of the Namdhari Sikhs, also enriched my knowledge and experience. Being a firm believer in healing and natural forms of medicine, he challenged me with complicated medical cases for which I had always to find a solution. That tested my knowledge and made me firmly believe that health is governed by natural laws and to restore it you have to simply rectify the faults and create a suitable environment. My work with polio children amongst his community created the basis for my rehabilitation programme which I used later for a research project in London.

I left India for Hong Kong in 1989 when my Centre for Integrated Medicine in Delhi was forceably shut by the local housing association on the grounds that the communal lift was used by my patients all day long. I suspect it was jealousy of my success rather than a financial consideration. In Hong Kong a chance participation in a radio talk show hosted by Aileen Bridgewater led to my overnight popularity there. It was followed by my diagnosis of a French businessman's tumour in his kidney through iridology which ultimately saved his life. This firmly established my credibility and within months I had a full practice, just as in Delhi. I wasn't a registered doctor in Hong Kong so by law I could not prescribe any medicine but I developed a unique skill in treating complicated ailments by using simple remedies or lifestyle programmes.

An offer to set up a Department of Integrated Medicine in London brought me here in 1991. I joined the Hale Clinic where I worked very hard to establish my practice. My patients helped by spreading the news about my work. In 1992, by coincidence, I met

Prince Charles at a reception and that meeting became a major turning point in my life. I knew then that Integrated Medicine, a name that I had created some 20 years ago, was to become a reality. His continuous help and encouragement saw me through various difficulties, both professional and personal. With his kind help I carried out my first research project on stroke rehabilitation with Marma, an ancient Indian physical therapy, at the Hammersmith Hospital. I opened the Integrated Medical Centre in London in 1998 with a team of 15 doctors and therapists. It has grown into a respectable medical institution catering to people from all walks of life, from both the UK and abroad.

I believe the time is now ripe to write about my philosophy, how I treat and prevent illnesses but above all about restoring health. I hope you enjoy reading it and practise what you learn.

Dr Mosaraf Ali
December 2000

ST. JAMES'S PALACE

This book is a (very) welcome addition to the now rapidly growing wealth of advice and guidance available to those who are interested in the process of managing their own health.

Good health is obviously of enormous importance to each of us, and to the nation as a whole. Ill health, on the other hand, is a costly business and it must surely help to learn how best to prevent it. It certainly makes sense to employ all the medical knowledge and skills available to us, not only from orthodox western medicine, which has achieved wonders, of course, over the last 100 years, but also from other traditions and sources drawn from many different cultures.

In the 'Integrated Health Bible', Dr Ali describes how to integrate conventional, complementary and traditional medicine into a lifestyle programme based on his experience gathered over 20 years, and developed more recently at his Integrated Medical Centre.

I am wholly convinced that the integrated health approach has the power to really make an immense difference to many peoples lives and to our society as a whole.

Integrated healthcare is based on the recognition of the uniqueness of each individual. It is about developing a healthcare approach, which takes full account of the unique physical, mental and spiritual make-up of each person, in the context of the environment in which they live. Most important of all, it is about encouraging each of us to take more responsibility for our own health, as an integral part of the management of our own lives.

To enable people to do this in the most effective way possible, they need help and support in channelling their own wealth of inner resources to aid healing. They also need information about, and access to, the wide range of healthcare therapies available. These, to my mind, can sometimes be more effective and less distressing for an individual than sole reliance on conventional treatment. Dr. Ali explains how the body is part of nature which is formed by universal rules and that any attempts to isolate man from nature can have serious effects on our health and wellbeing. He also explains how in a large number of instances the body knows how to heal itself when in crisis, given some assistance, and does not necessarily require intervention.

Therefore it seems to me that the further we can develop and integrate our approaches to health, the better it will be for us, both as individuals and as members of our communities. Dr. Ali has done us a great service in pointing out the way forward during the coming century and I hope that his "Integrated Health Bible" will help to revolutionize many people's lives and re-integrate mind, body and spirit.

The further we can develop and integrate our approaches to health the better, I believe, it will be for both of us as individuals and as members of our communities.

Part I
BACKGROUND

Chapter 1

WHAT IS INTEGRATED HEALTH?

Heart disease costs the USA $200 billion per year and is their number one killer disease. It is largely preventable under integrated health.

Integrated health is the gathering together of all the factors that contribute to your continued well-being and balancing them to enable you to attain your full potential all the time. This takes the form of preventive measures to ensure your maximum freedom from disease and adverse conditions; the most advantageous curative procedures in the event of your falling ill, using the best of all the traditional and conventional techniques; and optimising your condition to take advantage of your full potential.

I am a conventional doctor, who followed the normal syllabus, did a couple of years of postgraduate studies, and had the regular one-year internship. I have been in practice for over 20 years. That's all very usual. But in addition I have studied naturopathy, homeopathy, Indian traditional Unani and Ayurvedic medicine, traditional massage techniques, bone setting, Marma therapy and traditional Chinese medicine including acupuncture. I have mastered diagnosis through the pulse, iris and tongue – indeed, there are few forms of medicine in the world that I have not culled for their usefulness in these modern times. I am learning all the time.

Much of traditional medicine has been handed down from physician to physician and family to family for thousands of years. Its value lies in the wealth of experience gained over that time in harnessing the healing power of the body itself and empowering it to maintain health and correct imbalance caused by sickness. It was only some 300 years ago that medicine sought to employ science to bypass the practical experience that formed the basis of traditional medicine, and to provide an alternative which could be established quickly. Curiously the new medicine became known as 'conventional' and the old is now treated as an alternative, which has caused much confusion among patients and physicians alike. Traditional medicine remains the lifeblood of our profession.

I believe that there is much to be gained by combining all forms of medicine into an integrated whole, so gaining the best of all worlds. It is obvious to me that conventional medicine, as it is now known, has outstanding advantages for acute specific illnesses, while traditional and complementary medicine often outshine it when dealing with chronic ailments and conditions caused by a combination of factors (multifactorial conditions). Besides, modern technology has made conventional medicine cripplingly expensive and making the best use of traditional medicine may be the only way to sustain health services globally.

In my experience 80 per cent of everyday illnesses do not need the attention of a doctor. In order to release doctors from this unnecessary load and give them time to deal with complex cases the public needs to be well-informed on how to deal with these common ailments. That is the purpose of this book.

The power of the physis

First let me put medicine in perspective. Of the 6 billion people inhabiting this earth, between 50 per cent and 70 per cent, or probably over 3 billion, will go through their entire lives without any direct contact with a physician qualified in either conventional or traditional medicine. They will, in the main, lead full and reasonably healthy lives, those dying of starvation, malnutrition or epidemics, thereby creating headlines, being by far the minority. Another minority, living traditional lifestyles in Africa and the Himalayas will enjoy very long lives, often exceeding 100 years.

How can this be without access to medical help? The answer is simple. As Hippocrates, the father of medicine, pointed out 2,500 years ago we all have within us an unbelievably powerful health maintenance capability, which he called the *physis* (the root of *physiology* and *physiotherapy* – I pronounce it 'feesis'). This not only wards off or defeats disease but exercises control over every aspect of our health.

For example, from the moment of conception the physis of a mother looks after every stage of development of the foetus, normally without outside help, and masterminds the whole birth process, instigating muscular activity that may take place only once in a lifetime and yet is activated by most mothers (globally) with marvellous perfection, completely independently of any medical intervention. All doctors and nurses or midwives can do is supervise and make the mother comfortable, but in by far the majority of cases worldwide no doctors or qualified nurses are present. Even after the birth, the mother's physis retains an element of control by feeding the baby. By laying her hands on parts affected by colic, fever, anxiety, tantrums and so on, she reduces the baby's discomfort. This is a healing process recognised from time immemorial and actually taught to the medical students in the Institute in Moscow where I studied, but all too often scoffed at in the technology-driven world in which we live.

The extraordinary power of the physis is available and constantly active in every animal, including humans both male and female, and in most cases medicine takes the form of encouraging the physis to do its job. The surgeon removes a growth or sets a broken bone but leaves the physis to do most of the work by healing the injuries. Most of the drugs administered by physicians, conventional or traditional, provide the physis with the means to restore health. Indeed, most injuries and ailments, cuts, bruises, indigestion, headaches, colds, fevers, every viral invasion, are restored by the physis, completely independently and unaided. Every day we are inundated by germs and toxins we don't even know about because the physis, or its subsidiary the immune system, takes them all in its stride. Only if it is weakened by excessive stress, exertion, lack of sleep, lack of exercise, overindulgence or the like, do the defences of the physis fail.

I do not intend in any way to belittle the massive and extraordinary capabilities of conventional medicine, which have developed to an almost miraculous extent in the last 300 years, but it deals with a relatively small section of health maintenance and, I have to say, does it so expensively that it is hard to imagine that it can sustain its current drain on world resources. Indeed, its principle weakness – its high cost – has inadvertantly become its strength, in that money is power and the disproportionate budgets conventional medicine demands have led to disproportionate emphasis being given to it by governments. Furthermore, some governments spend billions of pounds on 'health care' and yet the health of those nations is no better than nations that spend far less. The extra money is not producing health. Traditional medicine on the other hand has proved itself effective and sustainable over thousands of years.

Conventional medicine has taken on the challenge of explaining everything about the body by science. It has made marvellous strides, but in so many ways has only scratched the surface. It may take a hundred years before it has fathomed the passwords and codes of the brain, the addressing of hormones, the dynamics of muscles or the secrets of memory. Traditional medicine on the other hand has never challenged Nature. It has always conceded that Nature knows all its own secrets and how to maintain itself. All we can do, all we need to do, is to help (like putting petrol and oil in a car, but leaving its maintenance to the expert).

Conventional and traditional medicine: learning to live together

I started my practice, having qualified in the conventional way, and quickly became aware of the perspective I have just described. The majority of the population of India, where I started practice, were well served by the traditional culture. When medical assistance was required it was available in the form of Ayurvedic or Unani physicians, whose university course incidentally lasts six years and is entirely comparable with a conventional course. The people who practised traditional medicine over the centuries were not amateur quacks as some would have us believe, but of an intellectual level equivalent to that of any conventional doctor, and they passed on their learning and expertise from generation to generation. The same could be said of Chinese traditional practitioners and these together provide the principal medical care today for a third of the world's population. To those who may try and brush this aside as 'third world', let me add that Japan and Hong Kong are in the forefront of modern civilisation yet they too have more traditional practitioners than conventional ones and have the highest territory-wide life expectancy in the world as well.

What conventional medicine has achieved in its brief 300 years of existence is to find treatments, partly for acute conditions that in the past have been beyond traditional techniques, but principally for those acute ailments created by modern society, such as new and more damaging toxins, and the terrible injuries resulting from crime, transportation accidents, warfare and industrial hazards. Traditional or complementary medicine can still, however, deal with chronic conditions, usually more effectively and cheaply than conventional medicine.

We therefore have a situation which is relatively new, where there are many different forms of medicine for different conditions, many of them recent developments, and competition has resulted in conflict and even professional warfare. This is a tragedy, and it has rested with just a few of us to try to redress the balance by adopting the opposite attitude of culling the best from every form of medicine and integrating it all for the benefit of the health of mankind and the cost-effectiveness of the health services.

Some may say that there are clear movements in the health service towards integrated medicine. Aromatherapy, for example, has been introduced in some hospitals, soothing music is provided, and acupuncture is used for pain relief instead of drugs. This is not integrated medicine. The complementary therapies are only used by conventional medicine where they offer no threat to existing practices, and then only as a 'feel-good' component. Some incidents have resulted in strong resistance on the part of conventional doctors to complementary therapies. For example, there was the case of the Chinese herbs that cured eczema, a disease for which there is no conventional cure. The herbalists in China Town in Soho, right in the heart of London, were flooded with patients when the news broke, some queuing up from 1 a.m. in the hope of obtaining relief. They didn't care about drug regulations, toxicity or illegal practice. They just went for it. The fact was it was a wonderful medicine and cured a lot of people.

The public demand was so overwhelming that the medical authorities set up a trial, in one of the major hospitals, on the use of Chinese herbs for the treatment of eczema. In order to protect the secret of the true ingredients for the cure of eczema, the Chinese herbalists blended together some 20 herbs and forms of mushrooms in one concoction, some certainly not necessary. The majority of the trial patients were cured, but some had liver damage. Nevertheless, eczema was a major problem and there was no cure in conventional medicine, except for steroid creams which merely suppress the rashes, so in the end the concoction was approved and prescribed under NHS licence. It was sold with a warning that there must be a liver function test before and after taking the product.

Now this is not unusual. Many drugs such as contraceptive pills, antibiotics used for acne treatment, hormone replacement therapy, high doses of vitamins, chemotherapy and anti-tubercular drugs are known to be toxic, some dangerously so, and are only used in conjunction with tests. When they cause illness, which they often do, such illness is known as iatrogenic – illness caused by doctors. Mostly, however, the doctors know that the body can normally cope. The physis (which they don't recognise) is up to it. Yet some conventional doctors remain totally opposed to the use of Chinese herbs to cure eczema because of the risk to the liver. The sad part is that in the hands of the traditional practitioners, who know how to take into account constitution and individuality, these herbs are perfectly safe and require no invasive tests.

Some say the position in the USA is better. There they are carrying out extensive tests on the healing capabilities of plants, mostly I suspect those that have been successfully and safely used by traditional practitioners for centuries. They even have clinics of 'integrative' medicine, where a patient goes before a panel, often a large panel, of different specialists, some of whom may practise complementary medicine, and the treatment is then a panel decision. This has three main limitations. First, it is limited to the available practitioners, for example there may be no exponent of marma therapy, by far the most efficacious treatment for stroke patients. Secondly it is very costly, occupying as it does the time of several specialists. Most of all it is bound by the limitations of conventional medicine, which is the controlling culture.

The shortcomings of conventional medicine

In order to understand some of the limitations of the conventional approach, we need to take a brief look at the history of medicine (a more detailed overview is given in Chapter 2). Back in Greek times diseases were categorised according to the organs they most affected. Pneumonia affected the lungs, gastritis the stomach, dermatitis the skin and so on. Centuries later when science had identified some of the pathogens, or agents of disease, the names took the form of bacterial dysentery, streptococcal/viral/fungal infection and so on. Later they started naming diseases after the person who discovered them, such as Parkinson's disease and Bell's palsy. Nowadays no new diseases are named. Everything is identified by syndromes, or sets of symptoms, such as acquired immunodeficiency syndrome (AIDS), Down's syndrome, chronic fatigue syndrome (CFS) and premenstrual syndrome (PMS). For example, CFS is characterised by fatigue, depression, muscle ache, memory loss, panic attacks, poor immune system, headaches, dizziness, digestive problems and so on (see Chapter 12). These symptoms originate from different organs and systems, including the brain, muscles, immune system, digestive system and circulatory system. This, therefore, is a clear example of how the entire body is involved in the disease process. It then became clear that this was true of most diseases. Common flu is characterised by lethargy, sore throat, runny nose, headache and poor appetite – symptoms with no apparent link to one another. It is a syndrome. Common diseases, even if focused on one organ, affect the whole body. Tonsillitis, appendicitis and tuberculosis are all syndromes, because some symptoms, such as fever, headaches, nausea and lethargy, go beyond the organs that are affected.

Of course this is how traditional practitioners have always identified diseases. Medicine has gone the full circle. But this evolution has had one devastating effect. The process of such categorisation over centuries has directed conventional medicine towards disease and away from health. No one has been able to categorise health, so it does not fit in with conventional medicine. Indeed, conventional medicine was originally directed exclusively towards treating symptoms (an allopathic approach), restricting the study of health, which had no symptoms to treat.

Another shortcoming of conventional medicine is the very science on which it is founded. From the period of the Renaissance, conventional medicine began to be studied in the light of chemistry, physics, mathematics, biochemistry, biophysics and all sorts of combinations of fundamental sciences. They studied it with scientific tools to establish figures and concrete facts. They started to measure everything: pH value of blood, blood count – all the constants in the body. Everything became figures and parameters. Everything was chemically analysed, physically recorded and mathematically calculated. So knowledge based on centuries of experience and observation got pushed aside and remained in the realm of traditional medicine.

There is so much about the body, however, that cannot be measured. For example, nothing about the mind can be measured. The result is that medical courses in physiology, the subject which originally was created to study the physis, does not these days cover anything to do with the mind. It goes as far as the way the nerve cells function, but the psychological or thought process is not included. At the anatomical level, students study the bone structure but not the detail of muscle function, yet muscles comprise over 60 per cent of the total weight of the body. Only in recent years has the task of studying muscles been taken up, in sports medicine. Again, you cannot measure the variations in people's constitutions, so this also is not studied and as a result hardly ever included in medical practice, though it is immensely important and one of the foundation stones of traditional practice. Conventional practitioners do, however, talk of blood groups A, B, AB and O, indicating that people do vary in their constitution.

This lack of individuality in conventional medicine limits diagnosis of disease. For example, doctors take a mean figure to represent all people, only occasionally recognising major differences such as male and female. The haemoglobin level in a healthy man is between 11.5 and 16.5. For women it is 10.5 to 13.5. Generally, however, if tests show the level to be within these ranges a patient is regarded as healthy and doctors will take no action on that count. Integrated medicine, however, takes the balance in individuals more seriously. A person is regarded as ill when he is found to be at variance with his constitutional norm, as has traditionally always been the case.

The battle for the body: sanogenetic and pathogenetic forces

Integrated medicine has to make certain concessions to conventional medicine in order that integration can take place. For example, modern medicine, only 300 years old, can scarcely be expected to accept 2,500-year-old concepts such as the physis. Integrated medicine has therefore put the concept into modern terms. While the agents of disease are called pathogens, integrated medicine now regards the power of health as sanogenetic (*sanos* – health, *genos* – growth). So in the body there are two equal and opposite forces interacting, sanogenetic powers (those that are trying to keep the body healthy by rectifying all the imbalances in the body) and pathogenetic powers (the elements that cause disease in the body by unbalancing it, the pathogens). So sanogenetic powers and pathogenetic powers are continuously struggling against each other in the body. In status quo you retain your health. If the sanogenetic powers are successfully working so that the pathogenetic powers are suppressed then the body remains healthy.

Let us examine this philosophy against a real situation. The skin is full of bacteria and yet it does not become infected unless cut or burned, thanks to its own sanogenetic powers. Every cubic millimetre of air is full of bacteria – germs – and even more so when travelling in a tube train or an aircraft. You are breathing in germs by the bucketful. So the pathogenetic powers are surrounding us. The food we eat is full of pathogenetic forces. If there were no sanogenetic counter-agents you would be ill, you could not survive. Take a normal meal, which might consist of nibbles such as nuts, a starter of fried food, alcohol, a main course – meat and vegetables – followed by dessert, tea or coffee and a piece of chocolate. You have blended some 15 different substances – chemicals – and dumped them into your stomach. Now you hope the stomach will sort it out. Each substance has different properties and they need different enzymes to digest them. If the sanogenetic powers were not functioning you would be in trouble. That's when disease sets in showing such symptoms as burping, acidity, digestive problems and bloating.

The sanogenetic powers are such that even if you misuse your digestive system, if you treat it like the municipal rubbish dump, you will usually be OK. But we take the sanogenetic forces for granted. We often do not realise what a tremendous load we put on the sanogenetic powers when we do this. After all, our bodies are our responsibility, but we misuse them, do no periodic maintenance, drive them to their limit, then go to the doctor, pass the responsibility over to him and expect him to put it right. You know what happens to your car or house, and your wallet, if you treat them like that. Would any executive or manager survive if that were the philosophy adopted?

Alternatively, we go out burning ourselves in the sun to get a tan, or we may indulge in chemical or drug abuse. The fact is we are continuously exposing ourselves to the pathogenetic powers that surround us, much of the time thoughtlessly and unnecessarily.

Now let us consider where the immune system fits into all this. The immune system is that part of the sanogenetic system that deals with warding off the bugs, the germs, the viruses, the fungi, the bacteria. The immune system involves lymphocytes (T-cells), antibodies (defensive bodies), lymph nodes, spleen, bone marrow etc. So, when external agents come into the body, the sanogenetic powers try to ward them off by sending out specific cells, certain chemicals or protein particles (antibodies) in the blood to destroy them. This represents the immune system in its classical sense.

The sanogenetic powers have many names. The Greek word was *physis*, which was regarded as the soul. The Indians called it *prana*. The Arabic word is *nafs*, which is equivalent to 'breath of life'. So physis has some spiritual connotation. The original study of physis was physiology (*logos* – study), so a physician was one who healed through the physis. Physiology was supposed to study the inner soul, the properties or qualities that God has given us, to keep our body and mind the way it should be.

The advent of science, however, caused medicine to direct study towards cells, tissues and systems, so that today in physiology there is no study of the mind, far less anything spiritual. It does not study why we do things, how we think, emote, transcend, exercise intuition or telepathic powers. It is like analysing the TV set or computer as a series of parts without considering the information flow through it.

When you say you are at your wits' end or exhausted it means you have come to a borderline state, in which sanogenetic and pathogenetic powers are in close conflict. If the pathogenetic forces are too great, if the stress is too great, perhaps because you have not slept for many nights, there is a breakdown; you get panic attacks, depression, obsessions, persecutions or even hallucinations. But the sanogenetic powers are there, even in the mind, trying to keep a balance.

The stronger the sanogenetic forces the better. You are healthier. Just as with two hand-wrestlers in a test of strength, if the arm of one contestant is tilted back by the opponent, it is then twice as difficult to get it back and go the other way. So if the sanogenetic forces are overcome, it is twice as difficult to get back to health. The forces need a lot of help. If you have given in, it is twice as hard. Similarly, if the sanogenetic forces are strong it is twice as difficult for the pathogenetic powers to force their way in. This is what healthy people achieve.

Approaches to treatment

Most people today are in the borderline phase, neither healthy nor sick. If you go to a doctor because you have flatulence he will say it is not a disease, nor is excess weight or insomnia. Likewise chronic fatigue or lethargy is not a disease. So the doctor will only treat certain symptoms, say, fever, diarrhoea, a cough, or tissue damage, but he will not go beyond that to rectify the cause which might have started the symptoms. Factors such as blood pressure, pH value, hormone level, temperature, urea level, red blood cells and white blood cells can all be measured. The body tries to keep them all in balance, within the acceptable range. The moment a blood test result goes outside the range, the doctors will take action. If it is within the range they don't consider the person to have any disease. But having constant parameters is no guarantee that the body is not under stress or is not on the verge of slipping into an illness. Disc degeneration or bulge starts long before backache starts, for example. The sanogenetic powers are weakened long before a viral infection begins. An intelligent physician, acting like a secret agent or a detective, will identify the telltale signs of a rapidly collapsing body and give warnings well before the symptoms manifest themselves. To such a doctor, fatigue, insomnia or malaise are all-too important symptoms. That's where integrated medicine comes to the fore. Prognosis or foretelling the advancement of health or disease is an important role of an integrated medical physician. He or she must know what the outcome of a 'borderline' state of health will be and warn the person in advance.

My philosophy is to work to keep people healthy and to serve those who fall sick by providing clinics with a gatekeeper. The gatekeeper should have exceptional diagnostic capability and familiarity with the whole range of medical resources. He or she will be supported by a team of qualified physicians (preferably doctors, but certainly people with qualifications of a level equivalent to a medical degree) trained in some branch of traditional or complementary therapy. Thus the full range of therapy will be made available.

In this book I will share my experience in integrating different forms of treatment and how they have a synergistic effect in curing acute and chronic diseases. Based on the belief that the sanogenetic powers in principle can override pathogenic processes, treatment is carried out with the person in mind. As will become obvious, we treat the 'diseased' before we treat the 'disease'. Once the sanogenetic forces are aroused, the body does its own job to expel the disease and restore health.

It is vital that the wonderful anti-pathogenic forces of medical science be integrated with the sanogenetic powers that traditional and complementary medicine strive to strengthen in the promotion of health, if we are to have a healthy, productive nation and a sustainable health (not just disease) service to provide health care safely, efficaciously and cost-effectively.

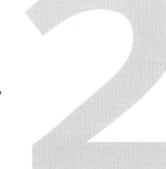

Chapter 2

THE HISTORY OF MEDICINE

The earliest recorded use of antibiotics was around 2700 BC when Egyptian physicians used to put mouldy bread (rich in antibiotics) on wounds. Chinese physicians were completely familiar with the circulatory system of the blood long before William Harvey disclosed it to Europe in 1628. When Fa Hsien visited Pataliputra (today's Patna) in northeast India in the fifth century AD he wrote of a civic hospital system where anybody, even the poorest, could be treated free of charge. Indian Ayurvedic medicine had by then been practised for a thousand years, so this form of medicine probably produced the first civic hospital system in the world. Clearly there is nothing new.

In order to understand integrated medicine, some familiarity with the fascinating history of medicine is necessary. Medicine almost certainly grew out of folk remedies that developed completely independently in different parts of the world. As evidence of this independence I would mention that the circulatory system was unknown to Indian (Ayurvedic) medicine until well after 1628 (when its workings were discovered in Europe), yet they had practised plastic surgery since the first century AD. In today's terms they had a different agenda. One needs to appreciate the way medicine has developed in different parts of the world and hence its strengths and weaknesses. The great value of integrated medicine lies in its culling the strengths of all other forms of medicine and putting aside their weaknesses.

CONVENTIONAL MEDICINE

What we now know as conventional or Western medicine had its beginings in Egypt, where physicians developed a good knowledge of anatomy because dissections were permitted. They were able to study physiology (the functioning of the living body), too, because one of the pharaohs allowed them to carry out the executions of condemned prisoners by dissecting them while they were still alive. This meant the functioning and structure of organs could be examined *in vivo*. They were also well endowed with plants and minerals and became knowledgeable in the use of antiseptics and preservatives, as evidenced by their success in mummification. Their records were excellent and much of their knowledge was written down. Alexandria became a centre of medical learning and many of the famous physicians from Greece and Rome travelled there to study. A devastating fire destroyed much of the magnificent library at Alexandria, but fortunately, by then, much of the learning had been transcribed.

Hippocrates

The history of medicine in all countries has been punctuated by the emergence of outstanding physicians. The first was Hippocrates, of whom little is known for certain. He lived in the latter half of the fifth century BC, and was a contemporary of Socrates. According to a biography written several hundred years after his death, he was born in 460 BC on Kos, a Greek island near Rhodes. Most of the accounts of his work seem to have been invented to suit the interests of the chroniclers. No contemporary statue, bust or written work by him has survived. More than a century after his death, however, a massive work, known as the *Hippocratic Corpus*, appeared in the great library of Alexandria, and although almost certainly a collection of many medical treatises, it is still regarded as a fair account of Hippocrates' work. Hippocrates has therefore, perhaps to some extent because of the mystery surrounding him, become an icon, the 'Father of Medicine'. His ethics are reflected in the oath still sworn by medical students on graduation.

His greatest achievement lies in the fact that he separated medicine from magic and religion. He stressed that disease was caused by the mental and physical state of the body and by environmental conditions. Therefore he looked for causes of disease both inside and outside the human body. He said that the purpose of medicine was to help the *physis* or natural healing power to cure the disease. He was the first person in antiquity to introduce the method of recording medical case histories.

He established the humoral theory in medicine, whereby it was believed that the human body or constitution consisted of four humours (blood, phlegm, yellow bile and black bile), and that people could be divided into four different constitutional types – sanguine, phlegmatic, choleric and melancholic – depending on which humour was in excess. Shakespeare was very fond of this classification and often referred to the humours. Othello was sanguine, hot and heady; Hamlet was melancholic, cold and full of pessimism; Lady Macbeth, calculating and cunning, a typical choleric; and Julius Caesar was phlegmatic, a balanced and composed personality.

Hippocrates' theory was that the humours are normally in equilibrium (health). But if, for example, an agent (bacteria or virus) attacks the respiratory tract then the body is in 'crisis'. One should help the physis or healing force of the body to eliminate it – by eating fresh fruit and vegetables and foodstuffs that reduce mucus, wearing warm clothes, inhaling to take the phlegm out, and getting plenty of rest. Cool showers should be used to bring down fever.

If the body's healing power failed to fight an infection within 4–7 days ('the critical phase' as Hippocrates called it) the disease entered the 'lysis stage'. Here medication was given, for example to eliminate phlegm. These were and still are the expectorants or cough mixtures which 'mature' the phlegm and expel it from the body, which then returns to its balanced state of the humours. The final stage was recuperation, rest and relaxation, on which Hippocrates placed great importance, but which is too often neglected today.

Hippocrates took great care in examining the patients and listening to their complaints. He always looked for a defect in the body's system or a cause in the environment. Thus if he realised that an ailment was caused by stress he would do everything either to eliminate the affliction by advice or counselling or to help the patient to cope with it. A person's diet was of foremost importance to him.

After his death, his son and son-in-law established a school of Dogmatism. In other words, teachings of Hippocrates were final and no new thoughts or development in medicine were possible for hundreds of years.

Galen

Galen was another great Greek physician, born in AD 129 at Pergamum, a great cultural centre of the period. From the age of 16 he travelled abroad, including Alexandria, studying medicine under great physicians and anatomists for 12 years. At 28 he returned to his home and was appointed as physician to the gladiators. In this capacity he gained experience of a whole range of physical injuries and wounds. He came into contact with internal tissue and organs, contact denied to others in his profession because of a ban on dissection.

In AD 162 Galen travelled to Rome, where medicine was flourishing and indeed had been extended throughout the Roman Empire. Archaeological discoveries have shown a remarkable grasp of herbal remedies and surgery, though the latter was somewhat limited by a lack of anaesthetics. Administering quantities of wine and narcotic drugs was about as close as they came to dulling the pain. The Romans, however, were very conscious of the deficiencies of medicine and adopted a policy of prevention above all. The famous baths with their massage facilities, the aqueducts and the sewers, as well as a good understanding of diet, were all part of a search for healthy living in an urban environment which was found to harbour disease by its very concentration of people.

Galen enjoyed a meteoric rise and was appointed as physician to the emperor, in fact he became the only physician in history who served three Roman emperors. He began to write about medicine and its philosophy. Hippocrates had separated medicine from philosophy some 550 years before, but Galen reunited them. This helped him in his argument against other physicians, whom he criticised to the core with crude language, calling them 'stupid and insane' if he did not agree with their methods of treatment or principles.

His knowledge of anatomy, built up over years of study and by careful observation of corpses, helped him to make many new anatomical discoveries. He had the capacity to integrate his knowledge of different aspects of medicine – philosophy, anatomy, physiology, surgery, and the role of the mind and the environment in disease. He was also a great diagnostician. His book *On Pulses for Beginners* included the first description in antiquity of pulse analysis. He pointed out that experienced pulse readers can detect an early stage of pregnancy in women, emotional states, the power of contraction of the heart, and the state of many other bodily functions. Until the mid-1930s all physicians, and some even later, were trained to analyse five qualities of the pulse – strength, volume, depth, width and frequency. With this information a skilful practitioner could judge the state of health and the body's ability to fight illness. Today such methods of investigation are often dismissed, especially by those who most advocate technological progress. Even the rate of pulse these days is recorded by pulse meter, helping to depersonalise medicine.

Galen's books contained marvellous diagrams, particularly of the eye, and his terminology for different parts of the eye is still used today: cornea, sclera, pupil, iris, and so on. The same can be said of diseases. Tonsillitis, appendicitis and pneumonia are just some examples of his terminology. He was close to discovering the circulatory system, only failing in his understanding of the link between the heart and the lungs. Of course, he had no contact with China.

Galen's authority was so lasting that, even as late as 1959, a certain Dr Haynes was summoned before the College of Physicians in London for having cast doubts on Galen's infallibility. He was readmitted to the College but only after a written repudiation of his former position.

After Galen's death Europe entered the dark ages. Medical therapy was limited to the clergy and confined to the expulsion of undesirable humours by purges (causing diarrhoea), emetics (to produce vomiting), cupping (using glass bulbs to suck toxins through the skin) or blood lettings. Medical progress virtually stood still on the command of the Church.

Avicenna

It was during this period that progressive medical thought shifted from Greece and other parts of Europe to Persia, Syria and other Middle Eastern countries. The works of Galen and Hippocrates were translated into Arabic and studied by the scholars. It is said that over 400,000 volumes of medical literature, all bound in leather, were kept in the library of Hakim II of Spain. Greek medical literature and knowledge that had filtered through via trade from Persia, China and India, and been translated into Arabic, combined with that which was available locally, helped the Arabic physicians to progress with research and writing. The greatest contribution came from Avicenna (980–1037), physician and philosopher, whose five-volume book *Canon of Medicine*, one of 276 books he wrote, has become the most famous medical book in the world.

Avicenna was a child prodigy and by 21 he had completed his medical studies and was well into practice carrying out his experiments. He was often called 'The Arabic Galen'. His principles were taught in Europe to medical students as late as the middle of the seventeenth century. The *Canon of Medicine* was truly the medical bible for almost 700 years.

In *Canon of Medicine* Avicenna not only expounded the humoral theory (see page 19), the concept of temperament or constitution, but also his experiments, medical recipes for different ailments and interesting case histories. In addition it has encyclopaedic details of all medical knowledge that existed before him. He described pulse diagnosis in great detail.

His work on epidemiology, in volume 4, was remarkable. He knew the pattern of outbreak of smallpox or cholera and controlled the spread of such infectious disease by segregating people. He definitely knew that smallpox was an airborne disease and that cholera was waterborne and therefore controlled them very well.

In this connection he wrote about hygiene, probably the first person in antiquity to do so in detail. He described how hospitals should be clean and airy with fountains, flowers and music. Like Hippocrates, he stressed the importance of pleasant surroundings in a hospital. I wish the hospital builders of today or the people who run them would read a part of what these ancient physicians spoke about. Very often healthy people fall sick just by being in a modern hospital. All you see now are arrows showing directions to different departments and overcrowding. Everything is matter-of-fact and practical. The healing humane touch is missing.

Avicenna wrote an entire book on cardiac drugs, as heart disease was common amongst people who indulged in rich food and did minimum exercise. Some of his prescriptions are still used today. The basic preparations used were raw silk cocoon, musk (a powerful cardiac tonic preparation obtained from the umbilicus of musk deer), mint, basil, ruby (stone) and aromatic oil. Many of these preparations have been individually studied in recent years by leading pharmacologists in India for their effectiveness. Today we may give cardiac drugs names like beta-blockers, cardiotonics, vasodilators, tranquillisers or diuretics, but the effects produced by the old drugs are identical.

Avicenna was the first person in antiquity to point out the role of emotions. He attributed the emotions to the heart and defined four emotions – joy, grief, anger and fear. A thousand years ago it was difficult for him to explain stress so he defined emotions that affected the heart because that is where they were felt. We know today that one of the main symptoms of depression is a 'sinking feeling in the heart' and there are so many expressions like 'the heart is boiling with rage', 'feeling heart-broken', 'sad at heart', 'heart freezing with fear', and so on, which show that people associate emotions with the heart because that is where they physically feel it (in the form of palpitation, missing beats, breathlessness, and so on).

Avicenna used to examine the urine, stools and even the smell of the body to analyse its chemical state. Today an experienced physician can detect high blood sugar from the smell of ketones – a nail-polish/varnish-like smell; or the function of the kidney from the smell of urea (the smell of decomposed urine in public urinals). From the smell of the breath one can analyse the state of digestion. Fermentation of carbohydrates will give breath a stale smell, while putrefaction, the decomposition of poorly digested meat or protein by bacteria, will produce a rotten ammonia smell on the breath. Thus body or mouth odour can give a physician clues about the state of metabolism or digestion in the body. Avicenna always liked to analyse the faeces and urine of people. He noticed that the urine of some people attracted ants. He therefore had it tasted (it doesn't say by whom) and these samples tasted sweet. He began to study these people with great enthusiasm and noted their symptoms down. He called the disease those people had *Zia bete* (*zia* – sugar , *bete* – wine) and thus the name 'diabetes' came into existence.

Avicenna gave details of massage therapy, methods of exercise, hot baths and steam or Turkish baths, as he believed in the physical therapies which aid the healing power of the body to repel disease. He also described the techniques of venesection (blood-letting) and cupping, and the use of leeches. The use of leeches has once again returned to medical practice. It has been found useful in the treatment of high blood pressure, polycythaemia (excess red corpuscles) and blood clots. Actually, there is a sound basis to blood letting. If a patient has a lot of toxins in the blood and half the blood is removed, this is replaced naturally by pure blood and the toxins are diluted by 50 per cent. Today leukaemia and blood cancers are treated using similar principles for removing unhealthy cells.

Avicenna put a lot of emphasis on diet and mode of eating. According to him drinks like water, juice and tea are just as important to health as food itself. He strongly recommended refraining from food and fasting from time to time to 'purify the blood' as this gave the body a chance to rectify itself.

Avicenna lived for only 57 years as he was killed in a war but in this short life span he studied and wrote enough to enlighten medical schools for almost 700 years. His teaching and philosophy were far ahead of his time. It is such a pity that medical students and the world as a whole know so little about this great man of medicine. His clinical studies and his sharp observation could beat any scientist of today. Yet it is sad to note that until recently only two of the five volumes of the *Canon of Medicine* had been translated into English. Much of his writings are in Arabic, Persian or Russian.

UNANI AND AYURVEDA: MEDICINE IN INDIA

So the position a thousand years ago was that medicine in Europe had been moribund for 700 years, but it had developed in Persia, particularly in the fields of herbal remedies, hygiene, humoral theory (where sickness is defined as a departure from the constitutional norm – an individual matter), surgery (by then they had better analgesic herbs), and patient care. By this time also Persian medicine had gained a firm hold in India, where it was given a new name, Unani, and established respect alongside the traditional Ayurvedic medicine.

Unani

Unani is the Graeco-Arabic system of medicine and Unani derives its name from the Arabic work 'Unan' meaning 'Ionia', a province in the eastern part of Greece. Ionian medicine was established by Hippocrates in 450 BC on the island of Kos. Hippocratic principles are deeply embeded in this form of medicine, one of the main principles being to help the physis (healing power) to heal the ailment. In his preachings Hippocrates clearly indicated that the majority of illnesses do not need medicines; instead, a perfect regime (diet, exercises, stress management, rest etc) alone can cure them.

Unani medicine categorises people into four constitutional types – sanguine (blood), phlegmatic (phlegm), choleric (yellow bile) and melancholic (black bile). Diagnosis is made by pulse reading, detailed questioning of the patients condition, examination of stools and urine.

Once the diagnosis is made, the imbalance in the body is corrected through a regimen of diet, exercise, physical therapy (cupping, massage, sauna) and medicines. The medicines used are herbal in origin and in exceptional cases gold and silver oxides are used (gold is used for the treatment of rheumatoid arthritis as in conventional medicine). It is also used for the treatment of irritable bowel syndrome, hepatitis, mild hypertension, eczema, psoriasis, leucoderma, infertility, chronic bronchitis etc.

Unani continues to be developed in India, where in 1998 there were 28,382 registered Unani practitioners, 100 fully staffed Unani hospitals and 867 dispensaries, 18 colleges (two offering postgraduate training) and 36 related institutes. They had published standards for 258 Unani herbal drugs.

Ayurveda

Ayurveda (*veda* – knowledge or science, *ayus* – longevity), the traditional Indian medicine, developed in a similar way, though independently. Again the emphasis was on health and prevention of sickness, acknowledging that this was infinitely preferable to getting sick. So Ayurveda tells us which substances, qualities and actions are life-enhancing and which are not. It comprises practical advice on cleaning teeth, diet, exercise and lifestyle for people in general, and detailed instruction for physicians on all aspects of diagnosis and treatment. Emphasis is on moderation and diversity.

Originally there was, no doubt, an abundance of folklore throughout India, which seems to have condensed into a unified system about the time of Hippocrates or up to a century earlier. This could be recorded and taught in schools and passed on through families. The icon of Ayurveda was **Dhanvantari**, about whom little is known, but his philosophy and practice is quoted by outstanding physicians and writers in the first century AD. **Charaka,** for example, is credited as the author of a compendium (rather like the *Hippocratic Corpus*) of 120 chapters listing over 600 drugs and laying down guidelines for physicians; **Sushruta** practised surgery and also wrote a book based on the teachings of Dhanvantari. He described inoculation in the form of introducing medicine through a scratch in the skin. Ayurveda developed an independent theory of humours or doshas, listing only three: wind (*vata*), choler (*pitta*), and phlegm (*kapha*). In all respects this theory was remarkably similar to the philosophy of Hippocrates and also emphasised the importance of taking a person's constitution into account in diagnosis and treatment. Ayurveda clearly recognised the process of metabolism and postulated a single energy source, *ojas*, derived from that process. A balance of the doshas indicated health, and imbalance was the characteristic of disease.

In about AD 600 **Vagbhata** produced a work of outstanding significance called *Heart of Medicine*. Some say it is comparable to Avicenna's *Canon*, and it was translated into several languages. He unified a mass of disordered and sometimes conflicting medical data. He described a seasonal regimen showing how activities should vary over the seasons and to what diseases the body is prone in each. He identified 107 reflex points on the body, reminiscent of acupuncture points, some of which he called lethal points or *marmas*, because puncturing them was usually lethal. This appears to have been linked to battle wounds, and advice is given on saving the victim's life. Later, martial arts practitioners developed this into a subject on its own, as further points were found which counteracted paralysis caused by blows to the *marmas*, rather like in Kung Fu, and it developed into a therapy for disabilities, marma therapy, which is still used today by a handful of practitioners in India and by my assistants.

In the fourteenth century **Sarngadhara** wrote quite a short compendium aimed at the general reader, rather like this book. It was very popular and can still be found in many libraries. The pharmaceutical industry used many of Sarngadhara's recipes during the twentieth century. He recorded for the first time many innovations, including the medical use of opium and the latest developments in inoculation.

Ayurveda is today the principal Indian approach to medicine and has government recognition. It is centred in Kerala and other states in the south, where there are many colleges, though there are many throughout India. Typically a degree course in Ayurveda takes four years (comparable with conventional medicine). Treatments and drugs are mostly standardised, though practice passed down from physician to physician still flourishes. The students study anatomy, physiology, pharmacology etc. just as medical students do.

TRADITIONAL CHINESE MEDICINE

Traditional Chinese Medicine (TCM) also developed independently. It has benefited over other forms of medicine from the fact that the Chinese used more permanent forms of writing and developed them much earlier than other cultures. For exampe, inscriptions on bone or tortoiseshell from the Shang Dynasty (from the sixteenth to the eleventh centuries BC) describe diseases of heart, head, intestines and stomach as well as epidemic diseases. Physicians were first mentioned in the Zhou *Book of Rites* between the eleventh century BC and 856 BC. By then they had identified seasonal diseases such as excessive dandruff in spring, scabies in summer, malaria in autumn and coughing in winter, which were treated with herbs. There were four forms of diagnosis: inspection, particularly of the tongue; auscultation (listening to the sounds of the patient's voice), breathing, coughing, belching and groaning (using bamboo tubes as stethoscopes); interrogation; and palpation or feeling the pulse. References to acupuncture, a procedure involving insertion and manipulation of needles at points all over the body, date back to around 2000 BC. One of the earliest discoveries was the analgesic properties of acupuncture, which gave Chinese physicians an enormous advantage over their contemporaries in surgery.

Hua Tuo was the most famous surgeon of the first century AD (Han Dynasty) and a master of internal medicine, surgery, gynaecology, paediatrics, acupuncture – almost every branch of medicine. Known as the 'miracle-working doctor', he was said to have performed many major operations, including abdominal section, using herbal anaesthesia. He attached importance to taking exercise and recommended therapeutic gymnastics called 'Frolic of Five Animals'. He held that smooth circulation of blood was imperative for health.

The oldest medical classic in China is called *Huangdi's Canon of Medicine*. The emperor Huangdi lived from 2698 to 2589 BC, but the Canon is thought to be a collection of many writings dating from that era, published during the Warring States period of 475 – 221 BC. This is more or less the time of Hippocrates and the *Hippocratic Corpus*. Over this period the Chinese developed a humoral theory based on four different fluids in the

The history of medicine

human body: blood, phlegm, bile and black fluid. They identified a central energy source, which they called *chi*, and they mapped its flow through the body by observing the distribution of the reflex points they used in acupuncture. They were very conscious of constitution and temperament and still to this day will prescribe different dosage and even different herbs according to constitution and temperament.

Wang Shuhe, who lived from about AD 210 to 285 (Jin Dynasty) wrote many books including *The Pulse Classic*, the first comprehensive book on pulse diagnosis still existing in China.

The Peaceful Holy Benevolent Prescriptions and the *Imperial Encyclopaedia of Medicine* were published between 960 and 1127, around the time of Avicenna. The first, compiled by **Wang Huaiyin**, included 16,834 prescriptions relating to various medical branches, with discussions on diagnosis and pathology of different diseases.

The Ming Dynasty (1368–1644) saw big developments in medical science. The greatest work at the time, issued in AD 1406 was the 168-volume *Prescriptions for Universal Relief* by **Teng Hong**, an encyclopaedia of internal medicine with 61,739 prescriptions and 239 illustrations.

MODERN MEDICINE

The extraordinary feature of all these major approaches to medicine is their similarity, despite their having developed completely independently. Their development of the humoral theory, with basically the same humours; the fact of a central source of energy, call it *prana* or *chi*; their development of the same forms of diagnosis, for example by reading the tongue and the pulse – how could this happen simultaneously, independently and in isolation, if there were no foundation for it? Yet conventional modern medicine has in the last half century discarded it almost entirely in favour of an approach that can give no prognosis of its long-term impact on the human race.

Remember that, at the time we are discussing, medicine in Europe had been moribund for around 1,300 years. With the advent of protestant religious movements medicine was liberalised around the sixteenth century, and with the development of natural science the medical profession, aware of its backward situation, looked to science and the promise offered by the techniques of prediction. Up till then all medicine had been based on experience and logic. However, people like Sir Isaac Newton (incidentally he was skilled in medicine), who was able to use mathematics to postulate the law of gravity and then predict the paths of the planets, saw the possibility of analysing the functions of the body and agents to such depth that they could predict the effect of chemicals and pathogens and hence circumvent the need for the huge amount of experience and knowledge built up in other forms of traditional medicine.

This vision took centuries to develop, indeed chemical drugs were not introduced into medicine to any extent until the twentieth century, and up to 1935 most pharmaceutical products were still herbal or mineral. Science, however, enabled a new branch of medicine to emerge, which became so good at treating acute conditions, hitherto non-existent or beyond the scope of traditional methods, that it swept public opinion and taxpayers' money before it in a flood of public confidence. It is only recently that disillusionment has crept in, through staggering statistics on iatrogenic (doctor-caused) diseases (a New England study revealed that 36 per cent of the patients in a general hospital had iatrogenic diseases), hospital accidents, medical errors which are said to kill up to 98,000 each year in the USA, unexpected serious side-effects of drugs (adverse reactions to prescription drugs are estimated to be killing 106,000 Americans each year according to the *Journal of the American Medical Association* in 1998) and hideous costs. People have begun to realise that the experience of centuries, indeed millennia, has a value they don't have to pay for. Of the utmost significance is the fact that insurance companies charge as much as 20 times more to indemnify a conventional doctor than they do a traditional practitioner. In defence of conventional medicine, one has to concede that it is relatively a very new approach to treatment and there are bound to be teething troubles.

Unhealthy conflict and competition has developed between traditional and conventional medicine, at the expense of public health. Now is the time, like never before, to realise that all approaches to treatment have their merits. We can enjoy life better, at less cost, if we cull the best out of all the immense work that has been done in the name of medicine and use it for the benefit of our health. This is the aim of integrated medicine and the target is a sustainable and safe integrated healthcare system.

Chapter 3

Hㅤow your body works

Physiology is derived from the Greek words *physis* (healing power) and *logos* (study of). It was originally intended to be the study of how the healing power or sanogenetic powers work within the body, but as time went by it became more and more obsessed with what could be proved by physical science, limiting itself to the functions of cells, tissues, organs and systems. It does not study how they interact with each other and what rules govern them.

Thus physiology gives detailed accounts of how the body's sanogenetic powers work and how the chemicals interact but does not talk about what controls the millions of reactions that take place. Physiology carefully avoids discussing the role of the conscious and the subconscious mind in controlling the various phenomena. It even ignores the psyche, the thought process, because it cannot be recorded. Every other function of the body is studied in detail. Therefore physiology is a distorted subject.

What makes the heart beat for the first time in the foetus to initiate the life process? What makes people different from each other or what determines the constitution of a person? What forces maintain homeostasis or equilibrium in the body? (Homeostasis creates constant body temperature, a steady heart rate, average blood pressure, standard blood counts, and constant parameters of blood.) These questions still remain unanswered, although science has desperately tried to explain them with its own tools. Until it does, logic is used to give general explanations, something that philosophers did for thousands of years before the sciences were used to study nature. Logic, however, is no longer accepted as a valid tool for proof and argument. Many things in physiology thus remain unanswered because science wants everything recorded.

PHYSIOLOGY

Let us examine some of the systems of the human body and look at some of the intriguing things that go on. The body is composed of cells, tiny organisms that are the smallest form of life. They float in interstitial fluid, the lymphatic fluid, which permeates the body, but because of their strong interaction the result appears to be solid, though highly flexible. Clusters of cells form tissues, which differ according to the function they perform, (muscle tissue and skin tissue, for example), and clusters of tissue form organs such as lungs and kidneys. Organs are connected into systems such as the circulatory system, respiratory system, nervous system and so on. (It is extremely significant, and I will come to this later, that the psychic system, or mind, is not included in a medical course on physiology.) Most cells replace themselves at intervals which can vary from a few days, as in the stomach lining, to four months, as in the blood, or rarely, as in the brain. Brain cells are provided with a huge surplus to compensate for the lack of regeneration.

The body owner, however, need only be concerned at this stage with the systems, and it is their functions that I am now going to run through.

The circulatory system

The blood circulation system must be taken first because all other systems depend upon it. If it fails you're dead. If it partially fails the affected section dies, becomes gangrenous and has to be cut out. It consists of a pump – the heart – main blood vessels or tubes known as arteries and veins, and minor blood vessels known as capillaries and sub-capillaries, thousands of kilometres of them, which make up the micro-circulatory network. During their journey through the body the minor blood vessels come into vital contact with the brain, the lungs, the liver, the kidneys, the skin and other organs. This system is the parameter of life, the core of sanogenetic power, the foundation of health.

The heart is no ordinary pump. It is so critical to life that it is basically independent of all other organs of the body, even the brain. During a transplant operation the new heart continues contracting while in transit. In the body it draws chemicals from the blood it pumps, uses them to generate electricity, rather like a battery, and sends impulses of that electricity to various parts of its own muscular formation to produce the pumping action. In the 1930s, radar engineers invented an electronic device they called a multivibrator which did the same thing. You put a battery across it and it just goes on electrically vibrating indefinitely without any other outside stimulus. When you see the output on a radar screen it is remarkably similar to what you see on a heart monitor in a hospital. The difference is that the electrical circuit in the heart has been functioning in mammals since beyond the mists of time.

Neither the heart nor the radar device are completely independent. External instructions, from the brain or a control panel, can cause them to speed up or go slower within limits. But if these external instructions stop, they go on working indefinitely at their own speed, which is why a patient can be conscious brain dead, but so long as the brain stem is functional it will go on and on and on. The doting relatives are left caressing only an independent pump, not a person.

The main blood vessels are the highways and byways of the circulatory map. They are well understood and well within the realms of science. They are also understood by their owners, who know that aerobic exercises develop the heart and improve the circulation. What is not so well known is that the micro-circulatory system is vastly different, and by far the most important, intelligent and complex part. The sub-capillaries are in such close contact with the organs they serve that they can act as trading posts, exchanging carbon dioxide for oxygen at the surface of the lungs and, when in contact with other tissues, delivering chemicals (proteins, energy molecules, hormones and enzymes to produce specific effects), white blood cells, oxygen, medicines and nutrients in exchange for toxins which they return to be eliminated. They deliver calcium to bones and insulin to the liver and muscles. How they know where to deliver oxygen or a hormone or a nutrient and how much, and whether to collect in return any of a number of toxins, and where to deliver them, is not well understood. It seems to be a bit like the Internet, where every packet of data has an address, supplied by a computer, which amazingly carries it across the world in a labyrinth of circuitry to reach a final destination along with millions of similar packets. This is just one area where the body is still far ahead of science. We do know, however, that aerobic exercises do little or nothing for the micro-circulatory system, which can only be influenced by constitution and lifestyle.

The respiratory system

The respiratory system is essential to the circulatory system because it supplies oxygen and removes carbon dioxide. It is also part of the body's cooling system and the power source behind the voice. It can remove some toxins such as alcohol during exhalation.

The average adult breathes in and out between 16 and 18 times a minute. The lungs have various defence mechanisms. In particular, the bronchial tubes are lined with tiny hairlike cilia which are in constant movement, sweeping germs, dirt and mucus out of your lungs. Tobacco smoke, however, slows down and actually paralyses the cilia. Dirt and germs that enter the lungs are then not removed and the mucus that collects in the lungs provides a fertile environment for the germs to multiply. This is why smokers get so many respiratory infections.

Breathing is one function of the subconscious brain that can also be controlled by the conscious. Thus you can hold your breath and regulate your breathing rate, slowing it down to calm the conscious mind. This is the basis of meditation. Yoga has dedicated an entire section to the practice of breathing. This is called 'Pranayama' and its main purpose is to calm the mind and oxygenate the body to improve its functions.

The musculo-skeletal system

Muscles constitute 60 per cent of body weight. There is more 'meat' in the body than bones. Yet the role of muscles has been neglected. For example, without muscles our skeletal system would not be able to support our body weight. An elephant when darted with chemicals that paralyse muscles collapses within minutes. It is a general misconception that the skeletal system supports our posture and keeps us erect. The fact is that the skeletal system only provides surfaces, for attachment of muscles, and joints to facilitate movement. It plays a secondary role in the maintenance of posture. The term skeleto-muscular system should in reality be called the musculo-skeletal system, giving priority to muscles. In addition to its role in movement and posture, the skeletal system protects organs (skull, rib cage, pelvis, etc.), facilitates blood synthesis (bone marrow) and stores calcium.

Bones have been studied very well, whereas muscles had been left under the charge of neurologists who study nerves along with muscles. Only recently has sports medicine begun to study muscles in detail. Specialists in this area have discovered new facts about muscles and their functioning. In the East, however, much has been done to study muscles. Every region (Thai, Chinese, Indian, Indonesian, etc.) has its own style of massage. Their physicians knew the importance of muscles for well-being and health.

The nervous system

The brain consists of trillions of nerve cells, each isolated from the other and yet exchanging information with the help of microfibres (dendrites) and neurotransmitting chemicals. The cells all over the brain are similar in structure and yet each one is coded to carry out a specific function. Some cells 'think', carrying out intellectual, logical and memory functions. Others 'feel' pain, heat, pressure and so on, while still others control movements. What makes them different is not known and, furthermore, what makes them carry out higher intellectual functions is even more of a mystery.

The brain's functions can be roughly divided into two types: (a) conscious, those of which we are aware, and (b) subconscious, those of which we are not aware. This should not be confused with the conscious and subconscious mind. When we look at a board displaying the timetable at the railway station, our conscious mind is focused on the train timing, destinations and so on. But the subconscious mind silently records everything else around us. Thus the announcements on the public address system, the sound of trains, the smell of coffee from a snack bar, the movement of people and the flashing of advertisement lights are all recorded into the subconscious.

Nature has divided the subconscious and the conscious brain in such a way that, where precision control is required, the former plays the major role. If the conscious brain were to attempt to control heartbeats or body temperature it would literally go berserk. These exacting tasks are beyond the capability of the conscious brain. Imagine using the conscious brain to command every muscle and co-ordinate them precisely in gait, writing or speech. It would be an impossible task, so the subconscious brain does that. The subconscious brain has been doing it for millions of years in evolutionary history. The conscious brain has evolved only recently and therefore has limited experience.

The brain is linked to the spinal cord, from which nerves, thousands of kilometres of them, radiate to all parts of the body. The voluntary nervous system controls the movement of our body – chewing, walking, urinating and so on. The involuntary nervous system is divided into two parts:

1 The sympathetic, or that part of us which controls our 'fight or flight' reactions. For example, in a stressful situation, the body needs to gear up its resources to face the situation. Therefore the heart rate, breathing rate, metabolism, body temperature, glucose absorption and so on go up. The body is on full alert.

2 The parasympathetic, which controls 'rest and repose'. The heart rate, breathing rate, metabolic rate and blood pressure go down. Digestion, movement of food through contraction of gut muscles, storage of glucose or fat, and so on accelerate.

The most miraculous thing about the nervous system is its precision. You can direct your limbs with marvellous accuracy. Imagine the co-ordination of all the muscular activity of a top table tennis player, all within minimal reaction time. Science doesn't know how it is done. It is a miracle worth defending against the enemy of a bad lifestyle. You can check this wonderful precision with your own eyesight, by looking at something very thin like an overhead cable or a piece of cotton or a full stop, and if you try and look from one side of its width to the other you find you can do it. Think of the minute movement of the eye in achieving this. It is possible because of the tremendously sensitive feedback system. The signal from the part of the brain that controls eyesight back to the muscles of the eye is as accurate as the finest machinery. The involuntary nervous system is carrying out complex functions such as this all the time.

Not all parts of the body have sensory nerves. The inside of the brain for example has no sense of feeling, so the cancer glioma can exist and grow undetected until it causes epilepsy or headaches by pressure. Bones have no nerves and can rot from the inside and you wouldn't know. Surprisingly the black centre of the eye has no nerves, and cataract operations used to be carried out by cutting into it with no more than a local anaesthetic. The white of the eye however is full of nerves and very sensitive, as a piece of grit in the eye is quick to tell you.

Clusters of nerves, as under the feet or ribs, have such a surplus of sensitivity that they are ticklish, and the pleasurable impulses produce laughter. Massaging in such areas, however, can be very beneficial.

It has been generally accepted that nerve fibres are specific to the job they are required to do, an assumption that suits science but not logic. Our nerves are known to grow very slowly, if at all, and I am convinced that treatment after surgery, for example, can divert signals through other back-up nerve fibres. I have met cases of loss of sensation after surgery such as sinus or face surgery, when I have been able to bring sensation back into the tissue by massage. I have seen it too in stroke rehabilitation, where I apply marma therapy, a reflex massage dating back to Indian martial arts. Here I have been able to achieve recovery of patients in a fraction of the time and cost required by normal physiotherapy, even under trial conditions in a London hospital. This would not be possible if signals in nerves could not be made to travel by a different route. If I am right, then medical science is still a long way off explaining the functioning of the nervous system and we should pay more attention to the logic of the traditional physician.

The hormonal system

Most vital systems in the body have back-up, and the distribution of hormones is a good example. Hormones can be transmitted rapidly through the blood system. For example, under stress the hormone adrenalin is secreted from the adrenal gland above the kidneys and distributed with a multi-address. It increases the heart rate, metabolic rate, breathing rate and body temperature, mobilises glucose and tones up muscles, preparing the body for 'fight or flight'. One hormone is producing 20 different responses and must be transmitted to 20 different addresses. The nervous system would have to use 20 different nerves to send the same messages so nature has thus created a more economic and effective way of doing this. The hormones travel rapidly through the circulatory system and reach their targets in a matter of seconds, allowing rapid multiple responses to be achieved.

The digestive system

Digestion starts in the mouth, where the teeth chew up food into particles and mix them with saliva. Saliva is alkaline and contains enzymes (proteins that speed up chemical processes such as digestion), in this case starting the digestion of carbohydrates. The mixture is then swallowed and transferred to the stomach, where more dedicated grinding takes place accompanied by secretion of acid and more enzymes. When the stomach has reduced the particle size to an acceptable level the pulp is transferred to the duodenum. This contains a fixed amount of bile, which is alkaline and neutralises the acid, and more enzymes to complete the digestive process. The digested mass then makes its way into the smaller intestine, some seven metres long, where most of the absorption of nutrients takes place, and then on through the larger intestine. Here water, minerals and the rest are either absorbed and the remainder is stored in the colon and bowel and then evacuated. Much of the lifestyle programme in integrated health is concerned with diet, because so many of the activities of the body depend on the efficiency of digestion. Too many people treat their stomachs as a municipal rubbish dump and suffer more than they realise.

The digestive system can be understood in the following way. The steel in a knife looks nothing like the earth it came from in the form of iron oxide, water, nickel and so on. Similarly human flesh is not the same as the vegetables, grains, meats and other things we eat. These are broken up into small bits by the digestive system and used as ingredients to synthesise different tissues of the body. Thus the basic building blocks – glucose, amino acids, fatty acids, minerals and vitamins present in what we eat and in what comprises the human body – are the same in both forms, but their permutations and combinations in each are different. Digestion and metabolism are the two main processes that convert one into the other. Briefly, digestion breaks up the food into units in the gut, while metabolism (assimilation) in the liver and other tissues builds what constitutes the body: blood, cells, storage material and so on.

The liver

There are over 200 functions of the liver. It is like a chemical factory and a warehouse. It is the next most intelligent organ of the body after the brain. It has two sources of blood supply. One is from arteries feeding the cells as in every other organ of the body. The other is from veins, arising from the intestines and transferring the nutrients absorbed from food. Therefore it has more blood than any other organ, holding as much as half a litre at a time. Nature has entrusted the liver with various functions, amongst which is the main task of detoxifying the blood.

If a tablespoonful of milk were injected into the bloodstream through a vein the patient would suffer acute shock and die within hours. The same milk when drunk goes through a chemical change, is detoxified by the liver and enters the main bloodstream as useful food material. Imagine if everything we ate or drank – coffee, soup, orange juice – entered the bloodstream without passing through the liver: the body would be poisoned instantly. The liver thus converts digested food substances into products useful to the body.

It metabolises carbohydrates, fat and protein into energy and stores them as well, discarding the waste. It produces glucose from glycogen when the body needs it, which is why when one is hungry one can put a sugar cube on the tongue and within a minute or two the hunger pangs are controlled. Try it. The taste buds on the tongue send a message via the brain to the liver to release a quantity of glucose to satisfy the appetite centre. Dextrose taken by athletes has the same effect. It isn't the dextrose that supplies the energy, it is the stimulated liver. Thus the liver stores glycogen in large quantities as a reserve source of energy. Similarly if the glucose content in the blood is high then this excess amount is stored in the liver as glycogen. Insulin is used as part of the conversion process. If the insulin level in the blood is low (as in diabetes), the excess glucose cannot be converted into glycogen and you get excess blood sugar. If, on the other hand, the blood sugar level really drops then the liver begins to synthesise glucose from protein. In other words, the liver is the main regulator of blood sugar.

The liver also regulates fat and synthesises up to 80 per cent of the cholesterol in the body. All the fatty acids that reach the liver are converted into fat or energy. When we take excess sugar and the liver cannot cope with it, or does not need it, then it also converts sugar into fat. So eating too much sugar can lead to fatty deposits in the body. The cholesterol that the liver synthesises helps build cells or is used to make hormones. The excess is either deposited in the walls of blood vessels to form the plaque that most heart patients dread or is converted into bile to be eliminated into the intestines. The liver therefore regulates the fat level in the blood.

Protein is another substance that is metabolised by the liver. It is first detoxified and then converted into carbohydrates or fat, to be used later as an energy source. Some is used to make blood, or to transport substances to the various tissues, such as iron to the bone marrow. Proteins are synthesised from amino acids, which are a by-product of animal or vegetable proteins in food.

The liver is also a warehouse. It stores various minerals and vitamins. It can store enough vitamin D to prevent its deficiency for about four months, sufficient vitamin A to last ten months and sufficient vitamin B^{12} to last for a year. Similarly iron and many trace elements such as zinc, magnesium and cobalt are stored in the liver. Eight of the 13 substances, or coagulating factors, that help the blood to clot if there is bleeding, are manufactured by the liver. Excessive bruising and blood clot formation in deep veins are symptoms of liver disorder.

Another feature of the liver is that it is the main organ that detoxifies and excretes poisons, drugs and hormones. If you took a course of antibiotics, four times a day for seven days, you would be accumulating a lot of it if you were not able to eliminate it on a continuous basis. Thus the liver eliminates the excess antibiotic and maintains the optimum level to destroy bacteria.

The immune system

This survey would be incomplete without mention of the immune system. 'Immune system' is a catch-all phrase to cover all the defence mechanisms of the body against agents that cause disease (pathogens). It is thus the only part of the sanogenetic forces of the body which attracts the attention of conventional (allopathic) medicine, and hence is often regarded by conventional physicians as the *only* sanogenetic force.

Pathogens range from a sharp stone which cuts the skin to a virus to a psychological threat such as criticism or stress. The immune system includes the clotting agents in the blood, mainly produced by the liver; the tonsils and cilia which protect the respiratory system; the lymph nodes; the white blood cells and antibodies in the bloodstream which attack bacteria and viruses; the spleen and bone marrow that produce cells that destroy invading bacteria or allergens; and some people would add the defence mechanisms of the mind – all unrelated. The only thing they all have in common is the energy source of the sanogenetic forces of the body, of which all the components of the immune system can be said to be a part. Hence any load on the main energy source, such as excessive physical activity, a test of endurance, concentrating at a desk or computer, undue stress, a drain on the adaptability of the body such as jet lag, failure to take a holiday or even a simple illness like a common cold, can deplete the energy resources available to the defences and holistically reduce their effectiveness until recovery is complete.

There is, therefore, no remedy that can be faithfully said to 'boost the immune system', only one that boosts the energy resources of the body. This might take the form of an improvement to lifestyle, such as diet, exercise, massage or meditation. Any claim that remedy X 'boosts the immune system' should be regarded with caution. At best it can only boost one component of the immune system and that may not be the component that you are targeting at that moment.

In conclusion, the immune system is the part of the sanogenetic force that is specialised to deal with the external threat from invading germs (living bodies) and particles (allergens and others – non-living bodies). Thus it is the Defence Ministry of the body with its intelligence agents (lymph nodes), soldiers (lymphocytes) and armament (antibodies, histamines) to destroy the invading agents.

Beyond understanding: the mystery of the body

There are many other systems of the body, some not yet fathomed, such as the reflex system that enables acupuncture to operate, the memory system and the power of the mind over the body. Science has not discovered how they work. The logic of the traditional physician, however, enables us in integrated medicine to accept the reality of acupuncture, memory and mind control and all the other phenomena that have been observed over the centuries and to get on and use them pending their scientific explanation. This is fundamental to my Lifestyle Programme which is designed to optimise all the systems I have just mentioned.

The body has its own intelligence and behaves like a system that is governed by laws of nature. That vital force that controls all the phenomena in nature (from geology to the flora and fauna) has its representation in the human body. These forces can be harnessed to a certain degree, but ultimately they act on their own accord.

I believe in this vital force because no science has been advanced enough to solve the mystery in its own language. At the moment it is beyond our comprehension. We can therefore apply general rules to support nature and specific rules to advance our understanding. The more we break up the body into smaller parts, however, the more difficult it is to understand its mystery. This argument is fundamental to understanding the philosophy behind integrated medicine.

Part II
OPTIMISING HEALTH

Chapter 4

Optimising Health

What is health? This is a question that has puzzled philosophers for thousands of years and to which even today there is no standard answer. Avicenna endorsed Galen's view that the body has three states. Health is a state that helps to maintain the functions of the human body through proper balance of its temperament and constitution in a sound and correct manner. Disease is that state of the human body which is contrary to health. Then there is a state in which there is neither health nor disease.

Where physicians over the ages have been absolutely clear, however, is about the importance of maintaining health to the highest possible degree, and this is still today the aim of integrated health, because the stronger the sanogenetic forces (see page 8) the greater the defence against the agents of disease that are pounding the body all the time.

WHAT IS HEALTH?

The difficulty in defining health is that, like well-being, it is abstract. With an abstract concept it is always difficult to draw boundaries. It's a bit like the emotions. For example, what do we mean by 'happy'? You can't measure it. Dizziness is not recordable.

You accept that it means that you feel unstable, as if everything is moving, but to what extent? In a severe case, such as vertigo, the whole world around you spins. It is an extension of dizziness. Likewise, fatigue is not a measurable condition. People say 'I'm very tired.' But how do you measure tiredness? People like putting figures on everything, to use a scale of one to ten. Then if someone asks how tired you feel, you can put a figure on it. But it is still subjective. It is the same with lethargy, depression, anxiety, and so on.

It is sometimes possible to explain what is happening. In the case of fatigue, for example, the muscles, the nervous system and the circulatory system of the body have reached the stage where they cannot respond to stimuli any further. You can see this in a simple experiment that students carry out at school. The leg of a dead frog can be kept contracting with nutrients and if you apply electrical impulses they will cause a reflex action. These movements are recorded as sharp peaks on a rotating drum attached to one leg. If you apply too many electrical impulses the reflex action will stop, but will return again after a period of rest. This is called the recovery period and it applies to all muscles, which have to replenish their energy before they can go on reacting to stimuli. In a human being this is what we call fatigue, but it is still not measurable.

Diseases, on the other hand, can be defined. You can list the symptoms, you can identify the syndrome. Very often you can isolate the pathogen or germ that is causing the disease. Not so with health, there are too many parameters.

Overloading the physis

Hippocrates and Galen spoke of the physis being in good condition when the body is healthy. Health suffers when the physis is overloaded. Let me illustrate the load on the physis this way. Consider a car. The electrical system is driven by the generator, a miniature power station. If the engine is switched off but the headlights, air conditioning and stereo are left on overnight, the battery will most probably be flat in the morning. So it is with the immune system, sharing its needs with all the other sanogenetic forces. If you load up the body with stress, strenuous exercise, bad diet, fluctuations in temperature and, like the car on a long journey, too little sleep, the immune system will cease to do its job and some of the billions of pathogens surrounding the body will invade and you will get sick. It is no one thing that has caused the sickness, but the total burden of a number of loads that have gone beyond the threshold of the immune system's capability.

You could cure the problem in the car, make it healthy, by a multifactorial approach of doing without the foglamp, adjusting the temperature of the air conditioner and reducing the speed of the wipers. Indeed, if you switch off everything except the engine the battery will charge up again – the recovery period – and the problem is solved. So it is with the immune system. No one load is causing the trouble. The cause is multifactorial. The cure is rest and, in the long term, moderation in all things and doing things to improve the energy level in the body.

Health is multifactorial too. It has many parameters, none of which can be measured scientifically, but all of which can be assessed reasonably objectively. Let's take an example. A young person spends hours every day at a computer. He takes no exercise. He grabs convenience food when he feels like it. He drinks sweet, fizzy drinks and coffee all the time. And out of the blue a friend says 'Come for a walk in the hills on Sunday'. So he joins him and within a short time he is exhausted, while his friend can go on walking all day. Yet if that young person were to be tested by his doctor he would find all his bodily constants (known as the homeostatic constants) within range. His temperature, blood pressure, pH level (acid/alkali balance) might all be at an acceptable level and his doctor would pronounce him healthy. What is the difference between him and his friend?

The health scale

Sickness is easier to define than health. The doctor will say a person is sick if any of the bodily constants are outside the normal range. Indeed it is quite easy to list levels of sickness, which medically can be defined in technical terms: off-colour, sick, seriously ill, terminally ill or about to die. Compare all the symptoms that amount to ill-health, but not enough to take you to the doctor because you know you are not actually sick. I am thinking of aches and pains, passing of wind, indigestion, dandruff, stiff and painful joints, dry, flaking skin or mild depression. Maybe you catch a cold or flu more than once a year. So it is possible to grade health in the same way as disease. For example a healthy person might be; off-colour, all right, fit, in great shape, bursting with energy or meeting his full potential. Notice that 'fit' comes fairly low down the scale. Since Roman times athletes have not been noted for their health, which often cracks up far too early in life. On the other hand a disabled person might be very healthy apart from his or her disability.

Now the first two levels on the scale, off-colour and all right, apply to most of us, I would go so far as to say to 80 per cent of the population. Indeed a high proportion of urban dwellers vary from alright to off-colour most of their lives. If they fall sick or seriously ill they know the 'health' service is there to deal with sickness and they will contact a doctor. Few, therefore, seek to rise above the borderline of health to become fit, or in great shape, or to be bursting with energy, or to meet their full potential. I suggest this is because conventional medicine has only recently accepted the existence of health as a positive state rather than just a lack of disease and as a result the administrations that largely finance it are focused on sickness and hospitals, and devote an unseemly small percentage of effort and resources to the maintenance and enhancement of health. Almost all governments misuse the word health to mean disease. The UK National Health Service is in fact the National Disease Service. This is one of the major reasons for its lack of sustainability. Major promotion of health would be far more cost-effective than setting out to cure preventable diseases. Think what you could do with the $200 billion per year that the USA spends on preventable heart disease!

Symptoms of health

So what are the symptoms or parameters of health? These have been identified for centuries in all forms of traditional medicine, which do focus a great deal of attention on health. Traditional Indian philosophy says that if you have an erect spine, a sound appetite, clear bowel movements eliminating all the toxins, sound sleep and clear eyes (to the observer), then you are healthy. When a person bounces into the room with an erect spine you know all his bones, nerves and muscles are in trim, his posture is good, he looks healthy. Stooping or slouching or avoiding eye contact is not healthy. If he has clear eyes it means that chemically his body is so good his eyes twinkle, absolutely crystal clear. Healthy people are self assured, have a sparkle, a spring in the step, shining hair, a firm handshake. You radiate all these things and people say 'What a healthy look'. Also you feel good.

If you feel lethargic and that you are dragging yourself along, if your posture is bad, if it takes a while to tone up your muscles, you are not healthy. (Don't worry too much about early morning stiffness though. This is quite common. If a few exercises put you right you may be completely healthy. This is particularly true of the elderly.) Feelings alone, however, are not reliable indicators of health. They can vary depending on your state of mind, your constitution, how you have hyped yourself up. Feelings can depend on the level of enjoyment and may not reflect health. The extreme example is euphoria, where someone feels great, but their body may be in a shambles and they could be about to die.

We could say that the lowest level of health is the absence of disease symptoms, no headache, no dizziness, no fatigue. This puts you on the lower borderline between health and sickness. But there should be positive symptoms, raising you up beyond the sickness borderline, where you can say, 'I am healthy. I am more than just free of disease'.

The main positive symptoms of health are: sufficient amount of energy, a feeling of being unrestricted, proper elimination, proper ingestion and digestion, sound sleep, ability to carry out duties without feeling strain or stress, a clear, focused mind, sharp short-term memory and recall, a body that heals very easily and can adapt to changes in atmosphere and weather, to travelling and to change of environment. (Travelling causes diseases mainly because it lowers the physis.) These symptoms are mainly subjective. They are our alternatives to the measurements of health, the homeostatic constants I mentioned opposite.

Symptoms of 'feeling even better' or 'meeting your full potential' include being constitutionally strong, having extremely good adaptability, rarely having symptoms of ill health in any form and excellent endurance. The cycles of endurance/tiredness will still be there but the periods of endurance get longer. Endurance is both physical and mental and is a critical factor when talking about super health. I am not referring to the marathon runner, though that is an obvious example, I am referring to the day-to-day stamina that is required to meet your full potential. Stamina is the ability to meet targets, to keep up the pressure. To achieve this level of health you have to do more than charge the battery. You have to look after it, top it up with water, keep the terminals clean, keep the rain off and so on. Incidentally, stamina is what fails first if you don't feel well. It is a telltale sign of approaching sickness.

A thousand years ago Avicenna had this to say about health:

'We can look upon ourselves in two ways, as a collection of chemicals and complex structures or as spiritual beings who need a body to make our existence complete. Whatever is the case, health is something we are born with and should be natural to us. So what has made us think that we have to make such an effort to create health? What happened on the way? To a certain extent health can be measured, by understanding the level of the physis in our system. Understanding the nature of physis can help to keep constant energy flow open, to keep a maintenance of our systems strong and we can call this healthy. We can learn to tap or unlock our inborn energies, learn the simple steps of how to maintain a healthy attitude. We can learn how to live in a fully honest and dedicated way, then focus will not be on weaknesses, but we will put forth our natural inborn abilities with ease and be free to enjoy the day and its activities more fully. Often we pass through a weakness without even noticing if we are happy with ourselves. Learning how to unblock the physis is one step in a natural direction and honestly sometimes an attention of love is the force that is required for a person to be able to recover.'

Factors that affect health

According to Unani medicine, as founded by Galen and Avicenna, the six essential causes of disease and the parameters that maintain health are:

- atmospheric air (if it is polluted or has germs in it that can cause disease)
- food and drink (what you eat and drink)
- physical or bodily movement and repose (how much you work and how much you rest. A lack of balance can cause trouble)
- mental or psychic movement and repose (how anxious or sad you are, how quickly you can return to a normal state of mind)
- sleep and wakefulness (if you don't sleep enough or too much)
- evacuation and retention (how much you retain in the body after digestion and how much you evacuate. The wrong balance can make you ill).

These factors essentially influence each other and every human body, and nobody can escape these factors so long as they are living. Avicenna also listed seven non-essential factors that can influence health:

- geographical conditions and other related matters. Other aspects of surroundings and environment, climate changes, changes of food
- residential conditions and related matters, housing, congestion, damp, air and sun
- occupation and related matters, type of work (repetitive strain, etc.)
- habits and related matters, indulgences, excesses, sports (need for moderation and diversity)
- age and related matters (certain ailments come at certain ages)
- sex and related matters (for example, women have gynaecological diseases)
- any other factor antagonistic to nature and bodily health (natural and artificial ionising radiation, electricity, geopathic stress from power cables, etc.).

These concepts were widely accepted by Hippocrates, Aristotle, Galen, Avicenna and all other followers.

How healthy do you want to be?

Each one of us has to ask ourselves some fundamental questions: do I want to be ill or healthy? Which is the more expensive? Which is the more enjoyable? If you decide to be healthy, then how healthy do you want to be?

Now this last can be a difficult question to answer because much 'enjoyment' is unhealthy. You have to weigh your lifestyle in the balance. But to help you answer the question let me make a suggestion. Take a ride on a commuter train around six or seven o'clock on a weekday evening. Watch the other passengers. Some will be sleeping, some dozing, some have eyes open but keep yawning, some are trying unsuccessfully to read and instead have a few sporadic comments to make as they are spoken to, others engage in animated conversation with their neighbours. How many are smiling or laughing? What about their posture: are they slouching or sitting erect? Are they fat or skinny or just right? How many have shining eyes? Who gives up their seat to an old lady? Remember, they have mostly had ten hours activity since they left home, yet they are so variable in their reaction to it. How would you like to appear to another observer like you?

THE LIFESTYLE PROGRAMME

If you decide to raise your level of health and lower your propensity to sickness, you will need to consider six factors: food, water, environment, sleep and waking, exercise and rest and the appetite and digestion.

To achieve this you need to adopt a regimen or lifestyle. This is the basis of integrated health. Over the years I have developed a **Lifestyle Programme** which is fundamental to my work. I use it as a preventive measure and also as the basis of all my treatment, when I refer to it as **Regimen Therapy**.

It is common sense that to keep healthy you have to eat well, sleep enough, do regular exercises, manage stress and maintain hygiene (cleaning teeth, going to the toilet regularly, washing regularly). This has been known to mankind since time immemorial. Hippocrates, when he talked about the role of the physis, clarified just this – that the strength of the physis can be maintained by adopting a certain lifestyle. Certainly it is common sense, though there is no scientific basis to prove it. We know it by intuition. Intuition, however, is an important aspect of our lives. We don't teach newborn babies to suckle the mother's breasts when they are born, they just do it. So the need for a sound lifestyle has come down to us from generation to generation and is instinctive.

The Integrated Health Lifestyle Programme is founded on these basic principles and rests on **a tripod: diet, exercise and massage. Moderation binds them together.** In ancient times, in the Greek healing temples, when a person was ill, the first thing the physician did was to put them on a diet, give them massage, rest and steam baths. All Greek and Roman baths provided massages, they had courtyards for exercises, pools for swimming, places to go to the toilet (these were always near the public baths, so people came in the morning and sat in rows chatting with each other – they didn't rush it). All these factors were regarded as very important over the centuries.

In the first century AD, Celsus, a Roman medical philosopher, wrote:

'A man in health, who is both vigorous and his own master, should be under no obligatory rules, and have no need, either for a medical attendant, or for a masseur or anointer. His kind of life should afford him variety; he should be now in the country, now in town, and more often about the farm; he should sail, hunt, rest sometimes, but more often take exercise. He should also show moderation in eating, drinking, exercise and sexual intercourse.'

Mankind has had plenty of time to evaluate the efficacy of such a lifestyle. What I have done is to make it practical to modern everyday life.

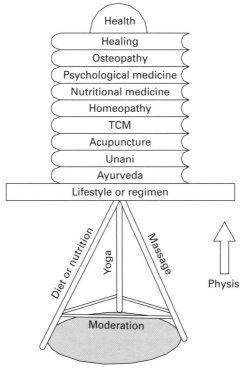

Health

Healing

Osteopathy

Psychological medicine

Nutritional medicine

Homeopathy

TCM

Acupuncture

Unani

Ayurveda

Lifestyle or regimen

Diet or nutrition

Yoga

Massage

Physis

Moderation

Disease

1 Diet

On diet, Galen, Hippocrates and Avicenna pointed out that we communicate with the world around us by absorbing food, air, water and radiation. So if the food (diet) is pure, the air is pure and the water is pure, then the body's cells and constituents will be pure. What you ingest goes directly into your system. Therefore diet forms a very important input. It has to be a diet that is suitable to the digestive process and to the availability of the digestive enzymes (you don't eat plastic because you can't digest it). Similarly stones, seeds and pips go right through the system without being digested. There is basically no harm in this but it does put great pressure on the stomach, which tries to churn them up. So we have to understand what goes into our system – what sort of water, food, air and so on.

2 Exercise

The next component is exercise, or more precisely the cycle of exercise and rest. Most forms of exercise are good, especially if you enjoy them. I have selected yoga as the preferred form of exercise because it encompasses both physical and mental stimuli.

Yoga not only exercises the body, but through the act of breathing it calms down the nervous system, it oxygenates the blood and tissues and it brings changes in the brain functions. It acts as a physical form of exercise and as a mental exercise and stimulant. So I have used yoga to cover both stress management and the Lifestyle Programme. By slowing down breathing you increase the heart rate. Thus yoga acts like an aerobic exercise, without need for jogging or running. I also advocate walking outdoors, which is very beneficial, enabling you to get your body going and take in air. Some amount of sport is essential, but if you can't do sport every day you should do some yoga. When travelling you may have to search for a place to do your sport and you need to take suitable clothes, whereas you can do yoga in your hotel room in your underclothes.

Rest is an important complement to exercise. Again this has been known for centuries: sound sleep, a siesta, periodic rest, a change of activity once a week and an annual holiday have all long been recognised as part of a healthy lifestyle. Indeed, the word 'recreation' means to re-create your physical and mental energy.

3 Massage

Massage has always been regarded as an important therapeutic part of lifestyle. More than 60 per cent of our body consists of muscles, which synthesise our energy and generate much of our heat. Massage stimulates these processes. Circulation is improved by massage. Also, touch has a healing effect. Reiki and massage by someone else are healing processes.

4 Moderation and diversity

Finally, moderation and diversity are pivotal to the Lifestyle Programme. Not too much and not too little of anything and a bit of everything that agrees with you. Small quantities of toxins can be handled by the body, but they each play their part in draining the body's sanogenetic powers. Take allergies. You may be slightly allergic to dust, mites, pollens and so on, but if the sum is less than the threshold you will get no reaction. In the hay fever season, however, there may be a high pollen count which takes you over the limit your body can tolerate. You may then get hay fever, or you might get asthma, eczema or any of the allergic reactions. Similarly, if the electrical load in the car (ignition, headlights, radio, windscreen wipers, etc.) is less than the generator's capacity, the battery is safe. But switch on the air conditioner and you are in trouble, not because of the air conditioner, but because of the total. So it is with the digestion or any of the body's functions. Load up one with toxins or over-exert the muscles and if that takes the total load above the threshold of the sanogenetic powers you have opened the door to disease. Moderation in every activity is the healthy course.

If you do all this you prepare the body, not only to combat illnesses, but to retain a certain amount of homeostasis or equilibrium, mental and physical. You are balancing your diet, circulation and mental processes. So diet, exercise, massage and moderation are very important. By following this regimen you are maintaining your machine.

It is also important even when somebody is ill. You have first to build up the physis, except in cases of accidents or bacterial invasion, where a direct agent can actually be tackled. For example, a fracture requires direct intervention. Ultimately, however, healing and recovery can only take place when the body participates. In a bacterial infection you give antibiotics, which supposedly destroy the bacteria, but actually you have only helped the healing process to do the rest of the job. The bacteria will have brought about other changes in the body which have to be corrected.

Over the next few chapters I am going to focus on the application of my Lifestyle Programme to optimising health. A summary of the key points is provided below.

Summary of Regimen Therapy

Diet

1 Avoid smoking and drinking alcohol.
2 Eat organic food, especially meat and poultry.
3 Avoid canned or preserved food totally – eat only fresh fruits and vegetables.
4 Avoid yeast-products, fried food, citrus fruits (except tangerines, clementines or oranges that have not been tampered with genetically), cheese, mushrooms, coffee, excess salt.
5 Balance your intake of fruit and vegetables with a sufficient quantity of proteins. If you are a vegetarian you should eat tofu, cottage cheese, soaked (for 24 hours) almonds, and sometimes protein supplements.
6 Drink carrot, celery, apple and ginger juice.
7 Drink a lot of water.
8 Sleep early and rest whenever possible. Do not take your body for granted and give it plenty of rest. An afternoon nap or siesta is very beneficial.
9 Dinner should be light and eaten early.

Massage

Have regular therapeutic massages with a focus on the neck and shoulders.

Exercises

Do daily yoga exercises.

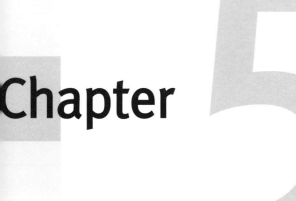

Chapter 5

DIET

A fit person can eat almost anything not actually poisonous, in almost any quantity, often late at night, particularly when they are young, and appear to get away with it. However, abuse of the digestion does affect health. Don't be misled by rugby players who feast and consume huge quantities of beer and yet appear to be in terrific shape on the playing field. There is a vast difference between fitness and health, a fact well known since Roman days. The purpose of this book is not to create athletes, who often don't enjoy long-term health, but to optimise the health of the average person by modifying their lifestyle. Vital to this is care of the digestive system.

THE DIGESTIVE SYSTEM

Teeth

Digestion starts when you take a bite of food. It is important to realise that if you have a problem with your teeth and gums you are going to have digestive problems. You must pay attention to your teeth and the way you chew your food. Teeth badly cared for are a source of toxins and a constant load on the liver. The state of your teeth, however, is between you and your dentist. I will deal with the chewing. If you chew your food well, you generally eat less and you reduce the load on the stomach. The primary digestion of carbohydrates that takes place in the mouth produces sugars (complex carbohydrates). These send messages to the brain saying that you are satisfied, so you feel satisfaction earlier. If you gulp down your food too fast, not only do you delay the feeling of satisfaction, you are also dumping unchewed food into the stomach. If you have unchewed or rough food such as nuts, crusts or seeds of different types, then the stomach is forced to churn it into a pulp because, unless it does so, finer digestion in the duodenum cannot take place.

The stomach

Now digestion in the stomach takes place in an acid medium, and the stomach keeps on producing acid until it has sufficiently reduced the size of the food particles. The longer it takes to do this, the more acid it produces. Furthermore, eating fast results in swallowing air which impairs digestion. Aerophagia, which blows up the stomach causes burping and indigestion, often leading to hiatus hernia. As soon as the air bubbles start coming out of the oesophagus they bring the acid with them and cause heartburn, sometimes even causing the acid and food to be regurgitated into the mouth. So, if you are in a hurry and gulp your food down, not only do you eat a lot more than you need before you feel satisfied, you create digestive problems. This is why it is very important to eat slowly.

Acid

The next part of the digestive process takes place in the duodenum. The liver secretes bile into the duodenum, creating an alkaline medium. While the stomach can secrete more acid through churning, the level of bile secretion is more or less constant. Now, the medium in the duodenum should be alkaline. If you have excess acid from the stomach it will neutralise the alkali, so the chances are the medium in the duodenum will be acidic rather than alkaline. Then the finer digestion will not take place and the food will remain there for a longer period, unless and until more bile is secreted. So, not chewing well, or taking substances which produce a lot of acid, can seriously disrupt digestion. Acid-producing foods include citrus fruits, vinegar, white wine and champagne, brandy, nuts, very spicy food, fried food, seeds, such as pinenuts or sunflower seeds, and food served at a very hot temperature. (If you drink hot tea, you get irritation in the stomach which causes extra secretion of acid.) Similarly, chewing tobacco or smoking nicotine can produce a lot of acid. Furthermore, as acid mixes with the alkali the reaction produces a lot of gas. This accumulates in the stomach. Up to five litres of gas can be absorbed daily, but more than this appears as wind. So people who have a lot of bloating and gas usually have it because of excess acid.

In short, for digestion to take place in the duodenum, the medium has to be alkaline. Excess acid will disrupt that, so chew food well and consume acid-producing foods sparingly.

Yeast

Another thing that impairs digestion nowadays is the presence of yeast. Yeast never used to be a problem. People used to take brewer's yeast as a supplement and eat yeast in bread. Yeast has only become a major problem because of the misuse of antibiotics over the past 40 years. Previously bacteria were stronger than fungi, but it was discovered that certain fungi secreted a toxin that could kill bacteria. Antibiotics, a fungal product, were then used to treat bacterial infection and fungi became all too powerful. This is why fungal infections are more common now than they used to be. Previously yeast would never cause an infection, it simply passed through the system. The body had a certain amount of immunity towards the fungus. Now that immunity is lost.

There are a lot of friendly bacteria in the gut. They are still there (though often reduced by antibiotics). But if there is a lot of yeast in the gut, or a mutant of yeast like candida, and it grows too strong, then it and the bacteria compete for food. Moreover, the candida being a mycelium, a type of fungus that has tentacles like mould, it drives its tentacles into the duodenum or intestinal walls, so that it can suck nutrients. Yeast has mutated because of the competition for food and takes another form to survive. As it sucks nutrients it makes the gut lining weak. Normally there is a barrier between the gut and the intestinal blood vessels, but when these mycelia create holes in the gut lining larger molecules of toxin, which should not normally be able to enter the bloodstream, are able to pass through. This is called the leaky gut syndrome. The molecules of toxin cause chronic fatigue and allergies. They are eliminated through allergic reactions like skin rash.

Another feature of yeast is that it brews its own alcohol in the gut. Anyone who has brewed wine knows that the formula is any vegetable or fruit, plus yeast, plus warmth plus sugar. The gut is an ideal environment, with a lot of carbohydrates, warmth, and plenty of yeast, so when you take sugar (the final ingredient) you begin to brew alcohol. Unfortunately it is an uncontrolled production of alcohol, a sort of illegal hooch. Instead of producing ethanol, the normal alcohol in drink, the yeast in the gut begins to produce butanol, propanol and other forms of alcohol, some of which are highly toxic to the body, especially to the liver. So you can have your own brewery in the gut. In fact, the digestive system is also a chemical factory, a warehouse, and the municipal rubbish dump, where fermentation and putrefaction (rotting of protein) can take place.

These forms of alcohol produce excessive lethargy. So people who eat sandwiches for lunch, full of yeast and carbohydrates, run the risk that one to two hours later they will begin to produce alcohol. Sometimes, perhaps surprisingly, the alcohol level can be so high in the bloodstream that people (including non-drinkers) become delirious, drowsy and are even sick. If airline pilots were to be checked for this they wouldn't be allowed to fly – the level can go that high. It would not show in breath, so car drivers might feel secure, but it could appear in a blood test, say after an accident. It might not show if the test were confined to ethanol, because it is methanol or propanol or some other form of alcohol, but the risk is there. It is, however, a temporary condition.

Bread, yeast extract, beer, soya sauce, many canned products, pitta bread and Indian nan contain yeast. So if you are not well and have problems of gas, lethargy after food, allergies or skin irritation, you should avoid yeast. People who don't suffer in this way, of course, can eat all the yeast they like. But in my opinion 80 per cent of people these days have gas or digestive problems. The moment they give up yeast they feel better. Antifungal products exist to kill yeast, but that is not the solution. If you have problems then your immunity to the yeast is weak.

Other factors can cause yeast growth. Bile is a natural suppressant of yeast overgrowth, so anything that reduces bile production or affects the liver, such as contraceptive pills, hormone replacement pills, and drugs that affect the liver in general, will reduce the bile secretion and can cause yeast growth. If you have too much acid in your food, it encourages yeast growth. So you need to cut down on your acid intake. Nowadays everyone produces enough acid because of the level of stress. Sugars feed the yeast resulting in a lot of bloating. So you should avoid excess sugar. Fructose, as in honey, is fine. You need a certain amount of carbohydrates but avoid excess. Other fungi, such as an excess of mushrooms or cheeses, can cause bloating, gas, allergies or sensitisation.

In short, if you suffer from bloating, lethargy after eating, allergies or skin irritation, control your acid intake and your consumption of yeast and other fungi. It is best not to take the risk and wait for fungus to be active. Just avoid yeast and fungal products whenever possible.

Other enemies of digestion

Coffee tenses you up. It produces general tension in muscles and constriction of blood vessels. Because of its cumulative effect you should not drink coffee regularly or in excess. Now and then is all right. But people should not drink it at the very time they do, namely when they are under stress. Coffee tenses you up more.

Watch desserts. As soon as you take sugar it suppresses the digestive process to some degree because the body senses digestion is complete. Try to avoid dessert at night, because that could keep the brain hyperactive and cause insomnia. Children who eat a lot of sugar are often hyperactive. The best time to eat fruit is between meals.

Fizzy water produces gas. It also causes problems with the digestion. Dairy products should also be watched. Many people have slight lactose intolerance. It can cause excessive bloating and production of mucus. Be sparing with canned products because of the preservatives, and with spicy, greasy, fried food.

WHAT CAN YOU EAT?

Remember the rule, moderation and variety. This gives you plenty of choice and an excellent menu. As a rule of thumb you need around 60 per cent carbohydrates, 25 per cent fats, 10–15 per cent proteins, various minerals and vitamins and plenty of fluids, at least 6–8 glasses of water a day.

Carbohydrates, fats and protein

Carbohydrates are the sugars and starches found in grain products, like cereals, bread, rice, pasta, fruit and vegetables. They provide energy to the body so it can carry out all its functions. Complex carbohydrates (unrefined sugars) are found in rice, noodles, yams, root crops, potatoes, bread, fresh fruits and juices, and vegetables. They are easily metabolised, though they take longer to digest than simple carbohydrates, and are cheap, tasty and satisfying. They are popular with athletes because they can be burned aerobically.

Saturated **fats** are contained in red meats, whole eggs, whole milk and milk products, and produce more cholesterol than unsaturated fats which are found in nuts and many vegetable oils. The body needs fats for a reserve source of energy, to regulate temperature and to cushion vital organs. Fats are a concentrated source of energy and contain vitamins A, D, E and K.

Proteins are the body's building blocks and they support growth and repair, help in digestion and feed the immune system. They are found mainly in meat, fish (grilled is best), milk products, eggs, soya beans and tofu. Nuts such as pecans, chestnuts, peanuts, cashew nuts and walnuts are a rich source of protein while they are tender (once the nuts harden the protein content is converted into carbohydrates). When seeds are soaked in water or begin to germinate, they convert their carbohydrate content into protein. This is why lentils soaked in water for 2–4 hours and seeds such as alfalfa sprouts, mung sprouts, wheatgerm, chickpeas and soaked almonds are also good sources of protein.

Vitamins

Vitamins are vital chemicals (derived from living matter) of which there should be an ample supply in a varied diet. Deficiencies, however, are serious. For example, lack of vitamin C causes scurvy, a serious skin condition. Lack of vitamin B causes beri beri, with changes in metabolism. Today such diseases are rare, but there are thousands of other changes that might take place in the body if there are vitamin deficiencies.

Beta-carotene (**Vitamin A**) counters oxidants and toxic wastes. Good supplies are to be found in carrots, broccoli, kale, peaches, apricots, watermelon and other green vegetables, as well as sources of fats. The recommended daily allowance (RDA) is 10,000

International Units (IU), which would be well exceeded by sensible helpings chosen from among the above foods. Taking vitamin A in supplement in excess is not recommended except by people who have been diagnosed as having a severe vitamin A deficiency.

Ascorbic acid (**Vitamin C**) guards against cell mutations and premature ageing and helps to prevent the oxidation of fatty foods. It is to be found in most vegetables and fruit, particularly broccoli, cauliflower, cabbage, kale, red and green peppers, potatoes, strawberries, citrus fruit and tomatoes. The RDA is 500 mg, which is easily obtained from the above foods. Indeed, a recent US study (see the Supplements section on page 52) recommends an upper limit from all sources of 2000 mg, exceeding which can damage the digestive system.

Cell membranes are fatty layers of which **Vitamin E** is the filling. It protects the fats from oxidation and soaks up free radicals. It also prolongs the life of red blood cells which have been exposed to ultra-violet light. It is to be found in foods providing fats, liver, green leafy vegetables, wheat germ, nuts, corn oil, soyabean oil and palm oil. The RDA is 400 mg. This amount may not be readily met because the foods containing vitamin E are not so popular. The US study referred to below recommends a maximum daily dose of 1,000 mg, an amount only obtainable through supplements. Exceeding this can increase the risk of stroke.

Minerals

Minerals are inorganic chemicals (derived from the earth) which in quite small but essential amounts support the formation of bone, nails, teeth and blood cells. Micro-elements such as cobalt, copper, zinc, selenium, and minerals such as calcium, iron and magnesium, are essential participants in different reactions, either directly or indirectly as catalysts to kick-start synthesis. Micro-elements form part of some 600 known enzymes that participate in the body's chemical reactions. If there is a deficiency in them there is bound to be an adverse change in the body's normal function. Any particular mineral can be harmful to the liver, pancreas and heart if taken in excess. Mineral supplements should be avoided unless your doctor has diagnosed a mineral deficiency. Remember, the liver stores most minerals for long periods. The most publicised minerals are calcium, to be found in abundance in many products, especially milk, and selenium the RDA of which is 55 mg and the upper limit 400 mg. People exceeding this amount could suffer toxic reactions. It can be found in seafood, liver, meat and grains.

Water

Water is required for all bodily functions, especially elimination, and to regulate body temperature. It needs to be replenished on a continuous basis. In addition to the water contained in many foods, the body needs at least six to eight glasses of water a day. There is no upper limit. Don't drink significantly with meals, it dilutes the digestive juices.

Water should be consumed every two hours or so throughout the day between meals. Other drinks have serious limitations. Alcohol suppresses the efficacy of the water it accompanies, as does coffee and to some extent tea. Most soft drinks and milk drinks are high in sugar that upset the diet regimen. Which brings me to the subject of weight.

Losing weight

1

Eat slowly. The more you chew your food the better the digestion. You also get an early sense of satisfaction as the carbohydrate digestion with saliva sends signals to the appetite centre to slow down.

2

Avoid acid foods. The more acid you take in the more quickly you want to eat because hunger pangs are caused by an excess of stomach acid.

3

Avoid alcohol.

4

Exercise regularly. Yoga, walking, swimming, aerobics etc. will cut fat by increasing the metabolism but will not build muscle bulk.

5

Avoid refined sugar, fatty or oily food, butter, cream etc.

Supplements

Supplements should be treated with caution. In April 2000 a report by the US National Academy of Sciences, (referred to in the sections on vitamins and minerals above), cast doubts on the benefits of taking large doses of vitamins and found no convincing evidence that taking large amounts of anti-oxidants such as vitamins C or E can reduce the risks of cancer, heart disease, diabetes, Alzheimer's or other chronic diseases. Previous research had found that excess beta-carotene can increase the risk of cancer in some people, especially smokers.

Today's food products, however, are different from their predecessors. In many cases the soil lacks the micro-elements we need. Thus today's fruit and vegetables tend not to be as potent as in the past, thanks to the use of fertilisers and other chemicals. Certain amounts of vitamins and minerals are essential to our bodies, so some supplements may be necessary. I do not see the logic behind large doses of them, especially when the body's absorption power is good. Moreover, continuous intake of any potent substance makes the body immune to it. One should therefore have gaps between the intake of vitamins for a month or so and take no more than you need. You could rotate them.

Menu-making

The traditional physicians used to categorise food as 'heating' or 'cooling'. In the East this is still done today. The terms are derived from the need to try to explain digestion in terms everyone could understand. Digestion was thought to be a process similar to cooking, so foods that promoted metabolism, or the conversion of food into energy, were described as 'heating' and those that slowed down metabolism were known as 'cooling'. Food can still be categorised in that way. To take a few at random, lamb, liver, chicken, eggs, asparagus, eggplant, green pepper, turnip, peach, rhubarb, banana, figs, thin grain rice, wheat, honey, and all sweet things, are 'heating', while beef, rabbit, fish, milk, margarine, lettuce, celery, sprouts, spinach, cabbage, cauliflower, broccoli, potato, carrot, cucumber, tomato, thick grain rice, peas, apple, melon, orange, tea, coffee and bitter things are 'cooling'.

The odd thing is that the English and American diet tends to be cooling (slows metabolism), while the oriental diet tends to be heating (promotes metabolism), which may be why there is such a clamour for Indian and Chinese food in Britain. My advice is to make sure you have a good balance of 'heating' foods in your diet.

You should bear in mind that different foods take different times to digest. For example, meat and fat can take up to four hours to digest (at least two hours), and most vegetables take up to two hours, while sugar and fruits are usually digested in one hour. Puréed food presents a greater surface area for the enzymes to work on and is therefore digested more quickly. Thus one should try to avoid eating food that takes a long time to digest, followed by food that takes a shorter time. The effect will be to block the already digested food from proceeding to absorption and it may putrefy before that can take place.

Breakfast should consist of fruits, yoghurt and cereals and perhaps some protein (eggs, cottage cheese, soaked almonds). Lunch should be substantial provided that there is time for an afternoon siesta or a nap of at least 30 minutes. Start with a salad, then with a protein (fish or chicken), vegetables and carbohydrate (rice, yeast-free bread, potato, pasta, yam, corn). Then eat a mildly sweetened pudding some 45 minutes after lunch. Dinner should be light unless eaten early (7-8 pm). It should not contain heavy proteins like beef or lamb, or spicy food as these take longer to digest. Dessert should be avoided at night.

When should you eat?

Lunch should be heavier than dinner, which should always be light. After a meal the entire digestive process takes place in the span of four hours or so. If you eat dinner late then the food particles remain undigested in the stomach and the process of digestion takes place in portions. Part of the food will be digested by, say, 11 p.m., another part by 3 a.m. Because you are not moving around, the requirements for food and energy are minimal at night. And yet you have dumped it in your digestive system. The food will be digested over a period of time. We are talking about double or treble (two-phase or three-phase) digestion. While you are lying in bed sleeping, the food stays there the whole night, is not utilised and causes maximum trouble. Most of the food gets absorbed unnecessarily. The body doesn't need it but it absorbs it. So most people who have large, late dinners will have weight problems.

During the day you work: breakfast gets utilised, lunch gets utilised, but dinner does not. Many people eat a light breakfast because they have had a heavy dinner and feel they can do without a morning meal. This is the wrong way round. Breakfast should be moderate. Lunch can be a good meal, but dinner is the one that causes problems with weight.

Tigers, when they overeat, let the food digest for a few hours and then throw up the rest, because all the left-over food is toxic. There is a form of yoga called Bagi, in which if you overeat you throw up. You let the food get digested for three hours and the rest you throw up. The Romans used to do this at feasts. I am not advocating bulimia as a way to get rid of consumed food, but rather that moderation and caution should be used.

Chapter 6

EXERCISE AND REST

The second pillar of my Lifestyle Programme is exercise and rest. As I explained on page 52, a combination of diet and exercise is the best method of weight control. In fact, this combination is beneficial for any function of the body.

YOGA

Yoga (*Yog* – union of mind, body and spirit) is an ancient Indian science. Through physical postures one obtains a harmony of the mind, body and spirit. Through breathing and concentration one brings tranquillity to the mind.

People have made yoga seem mystical, probably because it is the only form of exercise in which you control your breathing and get all sorts of unusual psychological and spiritual experiences. Whenever you try to control your breathing you are actually trying to control the subconscious part of your brain. In Kundalini yoga you can have bizarre experiences and movements of electrical currents in the body, especially along the spine from the lower chakra (plexus) up to the head. People practising Bhakti yoga can have out of body experiences and strange dreams. They experience changes in their psychic abilities and may become clairvoyant. Their perception (hearing, feeling etc.)

becomes heavily accentuated and they have powers to control functions of the body. For example, they can hold their breath for several minutes, slow down the pulse rate, change temperature, dull pain in the body; these autonomic functions are normally well beyond the control of the ordinary mind.

There are many different forms of yoga, but I use only one – Hatha yoga, which involves physical exercises and relaxation, and can be used as therapy on its own. Most of the exercises I recommend will shock classical osteopaths, chiropractors and even some physiotherapists. The movements involved are exactly the ones they think would cause 'disalignment' of the vertebrae and 'damage' to the neck. But these exercises have been practised in yoga for thousands of years. If they had produced any complications or side-effects, they would not have remained in use for such a long period of time. They are absolutely safe and these exercises have been thoroughly tested by myself and my staff on thousands of patients. They help to tone up the posture-maintaining muscles, and rotate and twist the joints and the vertebrae very naturally. (Turn to pages 64-73 for an explanation of how to do these exercises.)

Breathing

Breathing correctly requires training of the mind and the breathing muscles. This is where yoga comes into play. A special part of yoga is dedicated to the art of breathing. It is called 'Pranayama' (*Prana* – energy, life, air; *yama* – study, art). It asserts that the body and the mind cannot function properly if air is not exchanged in the lungs in a proper way.

Most people do not breath deeply and slowly enough. If you observe a child or a sleeping person you will see that during inhalation the abdomen blows out and during exhalation the opposite happens. This is the correct mode of breathing. If you do this, the rib cage expands and the dome of the diaphragm goes absolutely flat during inhalation. As a result, maximum air is brought into the lungs and the gaseous exchange can take place easily, leaving the blood enriched with oxygen. As you breathe out the rib cage collapses, the diaphragm is raised and the abdomen is sucked inwards. These three forces ensure that as much residual air as possible is expelled from the lungs. When people are stressed, they do the opposite, pulling the stomach in during inhalation and pushing it out while exhaling. It is amazing how most people breathe incorrectly either because of a general level of stress causing hyperventilation or because of habit.

After learning to use the breathing or respiratory muscles correctly, you have to learn to inhale and exhale properly through the nostrils. Nasal breathing is absolutely vital. The nostrils have hair. This hair acts as a filter for dust particles, allergens like pollen and other pollutants. Breathing through the mouth allows these particles directly into the lungs.

Near the bridge of the nose the nasal tract forms a dome and curves down into the throat, heading for the trachea or windpipe. The dome of the nasal tract is separated from the front of the brain by a thin bone called the ethmoidal bone. This bone is so thin that any blow to the nose can crack it. There is a theory that the passage of air molecules to and fro along the dome of the nasal tract creates a magnetic field that stimulates the frontal part (lobe) of the brain. This is possible because the separating ethmoidal bone is not only thin but highly porous. The frontal lobe of the brain is responsible for all thought process (remember the barbaric surgery called 'frontal lobotomy' to which schizophrenics were subjected in order to stop them from thinking?). Therefore, when the nasal breathing is stopped, perhaps by a heavy cold, there is a feeling of congestion in the front of the head. After 10–15 minutes of this, you may feel a dull headache at the front and experience some difficulty in concentrating. This has been observed in experiments. Therefore you should always try to breathe through the nostrils, even when talking, as this is beneficial to the brain.

It takes some practice to perfect the correct breathing technique. Slow, rhythmic, diaphragmatic breathing is ideal for better oxygenation of blood. The absorption of oxygen by the blood is determined by the level of carbon dioxide in it. Thus, if there is more carbon dioxide content in the blood, the exchange of this waste product with oxygen is more efficient. If you breathe rapidly you expel carbon dioxide and the blood cannot absorb oxygen efficiently. Thus hyperventilation (rapid, shallow breathing), as in a panic or asthma attack, leads to poor oxygenation of blood, which in turn may cause the sufferer to breathe even more rapidly. Yogic breathing with the help of the diaphragm is not strenuous and is the most efficient way to absorb maximum oxygen from the air.

Hatha yoga

Physical yoga, or the part of yoga that involves controlled bodily movement, is called Hatha yoga (*Ha* – meaning the sun, *tha* – meaning the moon in Sanskrit, the ancient Indian language). This yoga takes into account the bipolarity of all matters of the universe. There is a 'male' and 'female' or 'positive' and 'negative' aspect to everything that exists. Without this there would be no progress or development. If everything was the same in nature its machinery would fail to work and no movement would be possible. It is interesting that the Chinese, totally independently, derived an almost identical philosophy of *Yin* and *Yang*, so there is something in it.

Hatha yoga is designed to bring the 'right' and 'left' or 'hot' and 'cold' sides of the body into balance. In more scientific terms, the sympathetic and parasympathetic sides are brought into equilibrium. (See pages 27–29 for more information on the working of the nervous system.) It so happens that the sympathetic (fight or flight) responses take a predominant place during the day when one walks, works and reacts to the surrounding world. The parasympathetic nervous system (rest and repose) is more active at night when everybody needs to build, repair and prepare for elimination of waste products. It is perhaps for this reason that the ancient philosophers in India called this form of yoga 'Hatha yoga' ('sun and moon' or 'day and night').

Research

In the late 1960s a Soviet delegation went to India to study the effect of yoga on the human body and mind. In those days the co-operation in defence and science between the two countries was growing. The delegation included eminent doctors, surgeons, scientists, philosophers and a clinical psychologist, who were able to study yoga from different angles. They spent three months in India. They were first received at the Central Yoga Research Institute in Delhi. They examined the different aspects of yoga very minutely, studied various bodily functions and carried out numerous tests to see how the body responded to yoga. They were amazed at the findings.

In one experiment a yogi, connected to an electrocardiograph (ECG) was put in a coffin and buried. The scientists began to record the ECG readings of the buried yogi and noticed that within minutes the heart slowed down to a few beats per minute. Through the concentration of his mind he had slipped into hibernation, or *samadhi* as it is known in yoga. The scientists were absolutely baffled and they took turns to observe this phenomenon for six days and nights. Just before the stipulated time for unearthing the body, the heartbeats began to return slowly to a steady pace of 20 beats per minute. The coffin was removed and when the lid was opened the yogi was perfectly normal. Blood tests showed he had no significant changes. In India it is not unusual to see yogis standing on their heads with their heads buried in the sand for several minutes. You can see them showing off on Mumbai's beaches or in public places.

This experiment was filmed and stored in the archives in the Moscow Institute of Parapsychology, a secret organisation. The experiment proved that the conscious mind of a dedicated yogi can control breathing, heart rate, metabolic rate and the entire autonomous involuntary nervous system. Many practitioners can reduce their pulse rate to 40 beats per minute after meditation.

Advantages of yoga

Yoga helps to regulate the bodily functions and psychic processes, improves well-being and increases longevity. Compared to other forms of physical and mental exercise it has the following advantages:

1

Yoga improves oxygenation of the blood Oxygen is necessary for life and the various organs and systems function best when the oxygen supply to them is sufficient. The brain, the computer centre of the entire body, is highly vulnerable to low oxygen supply. If the brain cells do not receive oxygen for four minutes or so they 'die' or become incapacitated. (You know what happens to your computer if the power is interrupted for only a second.) If the oxygen supply is poor, they function with reduced power. The entire body then suffers a partial 'power failure' and the control systems are unable to function at full strength.

2

Yoga tones up the muscles of the entire body The various yoga postures are designed to contract or tone up different muscles of the body. There are exercises for the respiratory muscles, throat muscles, somatic (body) muscles, eye muscles, anal muscles and even the muscles of the tongue and face. Therefore yoga provides a very wide range of exercises. These can be used for therapeutic purposes as well. For example, someone who suffers from myopia (short-sightedness) can do the eye exercises and improve their vision. Many people with low-power spectacles have managed to dispense with them after doing the eye exercises. Yogic exercises are also preventive. For example, regular spinal exercises prevent backache, arthritis, fatigue, lethargy, weight gain etc.

3

Yoga produces reserves of energy Most energy is produced in our muscles. Vigorous exercises consume the energy that is held in reserve or actually produced during exercise. Yoga is gentle and therefore consumes only a fraction of the energy reserves in the muscles. As yoga oxygenates muscles, through gentle contraction and controlled breathing, a surplus amount of energy molecules is built up in the muscles. This invigorates them.

Normal exercises require a lot of oxygen for the muscles. Since the body's breathing cannot always supply enough oxygen to meet the demand in the muscles, some glucose is not fully broken down. A by-product of this incomplete combustion of glucose, called 'lactic acid', accumulates in the muscles causing spasms, 'knots', cramps and aches. In yoga, however, glucose is completely metabolised so such problems do not arise.

4

Yoga causes no injury to the body Yoga exercises take into account the body's natural movements. In fact, most of the poses are imitations of movements or postures of animals in nature. Thus you have cobra, cat, dog, turtle, monkey and lion poses. The limbs and parts of the body are stretched only as far as they can naturally endure and therefore the chances of injury to muscles, ligaments and bones are minimal. However, many types of injuries can result from forced exercises such as weightlifting or step machines and games like squash, tennis, golf, football and cricket provide numerous complications.

5

Yoga relaxes the mind Yoga is a mind–body integrating exercise and therefore the subtle movements relax the mind. Controlled breathing during the exercises keeps the mind calm. At the end of a session of Hatha yoga you are expected to breathe and relax in the 'corpse pose', thus ensuring that the body and mind are in harmony at the end of the session. Vigorous exercise, on the other hand, can sometimes agitate the mind – a bad game of tennis can leave the mind disturbed!

6

Yoga can affect the internal organs For example, yoga breathing exercises can clear the sinuses in case of sinusitis; they can open up the eustachian tubes and free the middle ear of infection and pain. Similarly there are exercises to help conditions such as constipation, flatulence, swellings in the feet, hypertension, poor appetite, insomnia, migraine, asthma and tonsillitis. Therefore yoga is therapeutic. Most other exercises are limited to one goal – cardiovascular or physical fitness. Therapeutic yoga, designed to cure ailments, is available at the Integrated Medical Centre.

7

Yoga exercises help to maintain good body posture In yoga the spine is the central axis around which the body is built. An erect spine creates an ideal situation for the body to function at its best. The nerves emerging out of the spine are best protected when the spine is erect and therefore all parts of the body receive proper impulses from the brain. Yoga exercises work on the spine from different angles. The spine is kept erect and the body is able to maintain perfect posture.

There are three main groups of muscles in the body: fast-twitching, slow-twitching and intermediate. The fast-twitching muscles can contract quickly and are fairly strong but become fatigued very quickly. Sprinters can run very fast but at the end of the race are completely exhausted. After a brief rest they can sprint again. Sprinters therefore have more fast-twitching muscle fibres. Boxers and weightlifters have a mixture of fast- and slow-twitching muscle fibres. Thus their muscles have both power and speed. Once fatigued, they take a longer time to regenerate their strength.

The body's posture is supported by slow-twitching muscle fibre which expands slowly and can remain like that for a long period of time without getting fatigued. Once it is fatigued, however, it takes a long time to recover. It needs a prolonged period of rest. A sentry can stand for up to eight hours without getting tired. But after that he needs several hours of rest to recuperate his energy to stand again. Bodybuilders can build up deposits of protein in slow-twitching muscle fibres through special diet and resistance exercises. These muscles do not have speed or power but have a lot of endurance. They can remain expanded or contracted for a long period of time without getting fatigued.

Yoga builds up these posture-maintaining, tolerant muscles. Yoga is therefore one of the best forms of exercise for the weight-bearing posture-maintaining muscles and is essential for the prevention of many spinal and other diseases.

8

Yoga exercises the mind through physical movements In achieving a yoga pose the body has to twist and turn in a complex way. Each movement involves the participation of the mind. For example, it is impossible to perform a head stand without concentration on the entire axis of the body. A person performing this pose has to imagine a force originating from the head and going through the spine to be released at the ankles. One has to feel the force pulling the heels or ankles against gravity and directed upwards. Without this participation of the mind a head stand is not possible.

The yoga posture 'salutation to the sun' is a series of complex movements and every step involves voluntary movements of the body. The stages of the exercise are not repetitive and so cannot be performed without the active participation of the mind. Thus yoga is a physical as well as mental exercise. The mind traces the movements and diverts itself from negative thoughts and worries.

9

Yoga improves circulation of blood and lymph In yoga, muscles contract rhythmically, aiding the pumping mechanism that helps lymph and blood to flow. There are various exercises that involve the raising of the legs and these help to improve blood flow through the veins to the heart. The diaphragmatic breathing also helps blood to flow back to the heart because a vacuum is created in the thoracic or lung chamber, forcing the blood to be sucked up from the lower limbs.

10

Yoga can massage large internal organs such as the intestines, uterus, liver and gall bladder. For example, there are several yoga exercises that use the abdominal muscles in such a way that the intestines can be massaged in a clockwise or anti-clockwise manner. There are other exercises that contract the upper part of the abdomen, thus massaging the organs there.

11

Kriya yoga uses saline water to cleanse the body Nostrils, stomach and rectum can be cleansed in this way but these are highly therapeutic procedures and need special training for performance. Cleansing breath is a method of expelling mucous, particles, nicotine, air pollutants etc. out of the bronchial tract.

12

Yoga has no age limit There always comes a point when age or infirmity demand that you give up aerobic forms of exercise. As often as not, that's when the rot sets in, unless you do yoga as well. You can go on practising yoga till your dying day – you never know, if you keep the breathing exercises going, it might not be your dying day.

One of my professors at university strongly believed that all psychosomatic diseases could be cured by yoga and meditation. He carried out a research project whereby he proved that stomach ulcers could be cured without medication by following yogic principles. This method of treatment involved simple cooked food, less meat, light dinners and regular yoga exercises. Amazingly, a group of patients who underwent this therapy had chronic ulcers cured in record time and without the use of any medication. He also had another group of people with hypertension put on a simple diet and regular yoga exercises with some meditation. All of them showed remarkable results and many were able to stop taking their medication.

Daily exercise

Though I have gone into some detail about yoga, by no means everyone will want or even need to become serious yogic practitioners. I do recommend, however, a few quite simple general yoga exercises be carried out each day. These are described on the following pages. They take about 15 minutes. Maybe I need to ask the question again: 'How healthy do you want to be?' Are you prepared to invest 15 minutes of your time each day in return for health? Do you ever have backache? Say goodbye to it. Do you lack the energy to see you through the day? Open the flood gates and take your fill. Does it take you half the morning to switch on? Do it in 15 minutes. Take it from me. These 15 minutes will be one of the best investments you will ever make.

YOGA EXERCISES

Daily exercise routine

Breathing exercises: B 1–6
Supine exercises: S1, S2, S3
Prone exercises: P1, P3, P4
Midway exercises: M2
Standing exercises: E3, E4

Breathing exercises

Stand erect for these exercises.

Cleansing breath

Normally when you breathe in and out you exchange about two-thirds of the total volume in the lungs. Besides this about 500 ml or one-third of the lung capacity of air is trapped in the passages and air pockets of the lungs. The lungs expand and contract, exchanging only the air that is inhaled. The air that is already present in the bronchial tube and in the actual lung tissue remains unexchanged. Cleansing breath forces most of this air out and brings a fresh portion into the lungs. This is a complete breath.

Before you start, blow your nose to clear the airway passages.

B1   **Cleansing breath 1**
   • Look up at the ceiling. With the help of your diaphragm, force the air out with a 'whoosh' (sniff out). You will breathe in automatically if you repeat this expulsion of air in quick succession – whoosh – whoosh – whoosh. Do this 15–20 times. As the air is expelled, the quick return of the diaphragm to its original resting position creates a negative pressure and brings air in with an equally quick and powerful inhalation.

B2   **Cleansing breath 2**
   • Look straight ahead and exhale forcefully, as in B1. Repeat this 15–20 times.

B3   **Cleansing breath 3**
   • Look at your feet and exhale forcefully, as in B1. Repeat 15–20 times.

B4 Cleansing breath 4
- Look to the right. Exhale forcefully.
- Look to the left. Exhale forcefully.
- Alternate between left and right and exhale on each side in succession.

B5 Cleansing breath 5
- Close your left nostril with the index finger of your right hand and exhale forcefully through the right nostril.
- Now close your right nostril with the thumb of the same hand and exhale forcefully through the left nostril.
- Repeat this 15–20 times, alternating between the left and right nostril.

B6 Relaxing breath
- Close your left nostril with your right index finger, breathe in through the right nostril very slowly, allowing your belly to blow out a little to create space for your diaphragm to descend and also to make room for the lungs to fill up with air to full capacity.

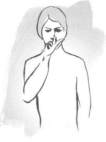

- Then close the right nostril with your right thumb and exhale very slowly through the left nostril, drawing your abdomen wall in and pushing the dome of the diaphragm high up to expel the air.

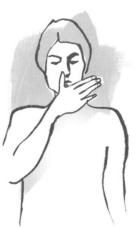

- Now inhale through your left nostril and exhale through the right nostril, closing the left nostril at the peak of inhalation.
- Repeat this cycle about five times.

Supine exercises

Perform these exercises lying flat on your back.

S1 **Child pose or pawan mukt**, sometimes called half-embryo or wind-releasing pose.
• Breathe in, bring your right knee to your chest, keep the left leg straight.
• Breathe out slowly, bringing your forehead to touch your knee.

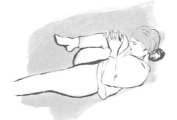

• Lower your head to the floor slowly, keeping your chin towards your neck and breathing in.
• Breathe out, relax arms and straighten leg.
• Repeat this with your other leg. Do this five times with each leg.

S2 **Supine twist**
• Extend arms at shoulder level.
• Bring knees up with feet on the floor.

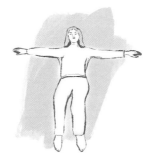

• Take a deep breath and turn your head to the left, while lowering your knees to the floor on the right (opposite direction).

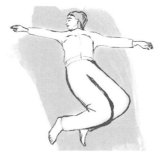

• Breathe out and then breathe in and out very gently. As you do this you must make sure that your shoulders are flat on the floor. You should feel the twist in your spine and your knees will gradually descend to the floor as muscular tension is released from the lower back.

• Repeat the exercise turning your head to the right and letting your knees come down to the floor on the left.

• Repeat two or three times on each side.

S3   Semi-bridge

• Put your arms by your sides.

• Bend your knees and bring your ankles back until they are directly below the knees, keeping your feet hip-distance apart.

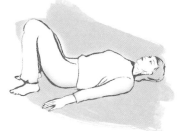

• Take a deep breath in and raise your pelvis as high as you can, tightening the gluteal region, and drawing your chin closer to your chest. You will feel a stretch in the back of your neck and upper back. Hold this position for five seconds. As you do this you will feel the blood rushing to your head and lower back.

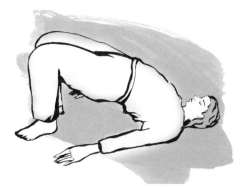

• Breathe out and return your spine to the floor, feeling each vertebra touch the floor as you do so.

• Repeat this pelvic tilt five times.

S4   Shavasana or Dead man's pose – deep relaxation

• Make sure your clothes are loose, close your eyes, put your arms to your sides and relax. Loosen up all the joints – shoulders, elbows, wrists, fingers, knees, ankles and toes – by gently moving them.

• Take a deep breath in, counting three (approximately three seconds), pause for three counts and breathe out very gently for six counts. Initially it will be difficult to maintain this rhythm of breathing and you may find yourself out of breath. If you persevere you will be able to acquire that rhythm. When you breathe in let the belly blow out and when you breathe out let the abdominal wall cave in, pushing the diaphragm out. For the first couple of days just practise the breathing technique until everything is smooth. The ratio between inhalation and exhalation times should be 1:2.

• When you have acquired the correct breathing pattern, try concentration. Concentrate on your forehead, on the spot between your eyebrows. Imagine that you are looking at an orange spot, the rising or sinking sun. Feel the warmth on your forehead. Divert this warmth to the top and the back of your skull and then to the sides and the temples. Imagine your brain relaxing and feeling warm. You can feel the thoughts, aches, pain, worries and stress simply evaporate. You feel your eyebrows relaxing and feeling warm. Next your eyelids feel light and relaxed. Your facial muscles and jaw muscles relax and feel warm.

• The back of your head feels warm and relaxed. Now your neck muscles feel warm and relaxed. Now your upper back feels warm and relaxed. Now your mid back feels warm and relaxed. Now your lower back feels warm and relaxed. Then your seat muscles, your thighs, your calves, your ankles and feet are relaxed. Experience the flow of warmth through these parts. You feel a gentle tingling sensation in your toes.

• Focus your attention back to the back of your head. Let the neck muscles feel warm and relaxed. This time let this sensation spread to the shoulders, the arms, elbows, forearms, wrists and to the tips of your fingers. Imagine that you feel a little tingling in the tips of the fingers.

• Repeat the whole process a few times, concentrating on the trunk and legs, shoulders and arms, until your entire body feels calm and relaxed. You feel light and almost weightless.

• Concentrate on your heart and imagine that it is slowing down. Imagine that all the blood vessels are dilating and your blood pressure is dropping. Your body should feel totally relaxed. You may by now be in a state of trance – neither awake nor asleep.

• When you have enjoyed this state of relaxation, return to your wakeful situation. Breathe in, pushing your abdomen out and breathe out, taking your abdomen in. Do this in the same rhythmic pattern as when you started. After a few repeats of this, gently open your eyes and absorb the sights and sounds of the world.

• After this exercise do not do anything excitable and remain calm. Your blood pressure may have dropped and you might feel slightly light-headed and a little cold due to the drop in the metabolic rate. Use a sheet to cover yourself while you do this exercise.

• This exercise should last for 15–20 minutes. Do not count time, just train your mind to do the exercise for this set time. Make sure that the door of your room is locked and the telephones are switched off. No one should disturb you while you do this. It is your 'prayer time', meant for your own relaxation and enlightenment.

Prone exercises

Lie flat on your stomach for these exercises.

P1   Cobra – full

• Place your palms flat on the floor beside your shoulders.

• Take a deep breath in, lift your torso up and look up to the ceiling. The entire body is arched back with the help of the back muscles and the arms give it minimal support.

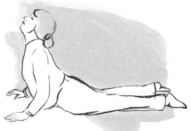

• Breathe out and gently return to the original position with forehead on the floor. Repeat this five times.

P2   Cobra – half

• Put your elbows by your sides. Take a deep breath in and raise your head looking up. Hold breath for five seconds and slowly come down, breathing out. The forehead should touch the floor. Repeat this five times.

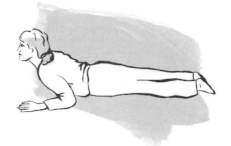

P3 **Self-traction**
- Lie down on your front on the floor.
- Put your hands together at the wrists and open your hands to make a bowl. Rest your chin on this bowl and place your palms on either side of your face. Your chin should rest firmly on the base of your palms.

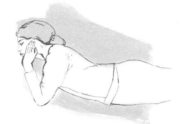

- Join your elbows together, push them slightly forward and start to look up, so that you feel a traction of the neck. Breathe in and out very gently. On doing this a stretch should be felt in your entire spine. Hold this position for a couple of minutes.

P4 **Swing**
- Put both arms by your sides with palms under your thighs.
- Take a deep breath in and raise your torso as well as your legs up in the air. Hold the breath in this position.
- Arch your back to look up and stretch your toes out. You should feel the tightness along the back muscles, the seat muscles and the hamstrings and calves. Hold this position for a count of five.

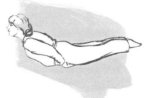

- Return to the normal position, breathing out again and placing your forehead on the floor. Repeat five times.

P5 **Swing – modified**
- Lie on your stomach and place both hands behind your back.
- Take a deep breath in, hold the breath and lift your torso up, raising your head and feet above the floor. Look as far up as you can and stretch out, as if someone is pulling your feet away.
- Stay in this position for five seconds and return to the original position, breathing out gently as you do so. Repeat this five times.

Midway exercises

M1   Squatting
• Sit on your ankles with knees bent, on the floor. Sit for two to three minutes.

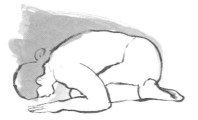

M2   Turtle pose
• Kneel and sit back on your heels. Place both elbows by the sides of the knees by bending forwards. Put your forehead on the floor.

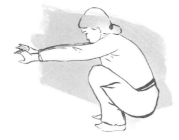

• Take a deep breath in and raise your head and look as far back as you can, keeping the elbows on the floor. Push your chest forwards. Hold your breath in this position for five seconds.

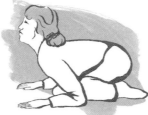

• Slowly breathe out and return to the original position. Repeat this five times.

M3   Spinal twist
• Sit upright on a chair or stool. Raise your elbows and clasp your hands in front of the chest.
• Breathe in as you twist to the right looking over your right shoulder. Breathe out slowly as you return to the original position.
• Do the same on the left. Repeat this five times.

Standing exercises

E1   Abdominal pump or bandhi
- Stand erect. Breathe in deep and then exhale deeply until you have expelled as much air as you can (even the residual air). Lean forward, looking straight ahead as you breathe out. While doing this draw the abdominal wall in.
- Then expand your abdomen and pull it in alternately. Make sure you 'hold' your breathing activity. Your belly should come out and then go right in as if to touch the rear part of the abdominal cavity. Repeat this five to ten times.

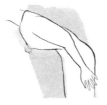

- Relax and breathe normally. This exercise tones up the muscles of the gut and bowels and improves circulation. It also massages the internal organs (gall bladder, pancreas and the heart).

E2   Abdominal massage
- Stand with feet apart. With one hand, rub deeply in a wide circular motion around your abdomen over the colon in a clockwise direction (to an observer in front of you) for about one minute.

E3   Arching back
- Stand with feet together. Tighten your seat muscles. Breathe in.
- Place both hands on your seat and push it forward. As you do this, look up, arching your back. Do not bend your knees while doing this. Hold your breath for five seconds and return to the original position on breathing out.

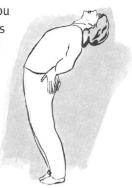

- Repeat this five times. You should be able to feel the tension in your lower back and the release of it when you return to the original position.

E4 Arms arch

• Stand with feet together. Take a deep breath in and hold your breath.

• Entwine your fingers behind your back, tighten your seat muscles and pull both arms down as if to touch your heels. Arch your back as you do this and look up. You should get the feeling that your back muscles and the muscles of your arms are taut.

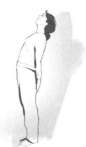

• Hold this position for a count of five. Breathe out and return to the normal position.

E5 Head roll

• Bend your head so that your chin touches your chest.

• Rotate your head in a clockwise direction, making sure that parts of your head (chin, lower jaw, back of head) touch your chest and shoulder throughout its journey. This way a total head roll is performed and the chances of dizziness are minimised.

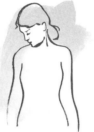

• Do this five times and repeat in the anticlockwise direction.

▪ This exercise will help to grind osteophytes or calcium deposits that so often settle on the joint surfaces all around. This releases the joints from stiffness.

E6 Neck twist

• Look ahead and grip your right shoulder with your left hand. Place the right arm behind your back.

• Take a deep breath in and rotate your head towards the right, while simultaneously pulling your right shoulder forward with your left hand. Hold your breath for five seconds. By doing this you will feel the stretch in the muscles of the right side of your neck and a release of tension in its joints.

• Return to the original position. Repeat the same with the other side. Do this five times in each direction.

▪ This exercise will strengthen the muscles of your neck and improve the movement of your neck in both directions, releasing the stiffness and shifting vertebrae that are out of alignment back into their original position. This often acts like a self-manipulation.

OTHER EXERCISE

Of course there are many other excellent forms of exercise and I would like to say a few words about **walking**. One of my regular projects is to take patients on walking trips in the Himalayas. Many have been seriously ill with chronic fatigue syndrome, ME, nervous disorders, various stages of paralysis, bereavement, and so on. Mainly they suffer from severe stress-related illnesses. The transformation during two weeks of trekking is astounding. They can all walk, young or old and however sick. So can you. Here are some of the benefits of walking: it helps to improve blood circulation, it helps to restore joint mobility and reduces joint pain, toxins are eliminated through perspiration, the brain gets fresh oxygen, the digestion is improved, lung capacity and function are improved, it improves posture, it disperses feelings of tiredness and lethargy, walking on green grass improves eyesight, it restores the body's equilibrium, it helps reduce weight, it reduces high blood pressure, it improves the skin condition, it reduces stress and tension, and it has a beneficial effect on diabetes. Like yoga, it has no age limit. One of the reasons villagers are more healthy than urban dwellers is that they walk a lot. So get on out there and walk, walk, walk.

REST

The body needs rest at diverse intervals because of the different recovery periods of the various tissues. This is one of the few aspects of traditional behaviour with which most people agree, though some disregard it. All mammals sleep at least once in 24 hours and humans tend to sleep at night, traditionally for about eight hours, though it is a recorded fact of modern society that this has now been reduced to about six hours on average for adults. Make sure your sleep is sound (you can find out more about sleep and sleep disorders on pages 216–226). From time immemorial people have rested, or adopted a complete change of behaviour once a week. It is also traditional to take a holiday once a year. Make sure all these are resting. Avoid working, or celebrating, into the night. Avoid working at weekends. Don't go on holiday so stressed out it takes you the whole time to recover. Give yourself a chance to enjoy your holidays. Your body is built to require periodic recovery periods and you disregard these at your peril, though the penalties do not always occur at the time. The damage to your body more often appears later in life, when you sit in your wheelchair muttering 'If only ...'

Relaxation is important. In some of your rest periods try to achieve total relaxation (see Shavasana (S4) in the yoga exercises). Ten to twenty minutes doing this each day will work wonders in stress management.

Meditation

Relaxation is the first step to meditation. This is not an integral part of my Lifestyle Programme, but I do recommend it to patients whose condition could benefit from it. However, healthy people do adopt it as part of their lifestyle because of its special benefits in stress management and mind control, which can be developed to the point where conscious and subconscious become interactive and parapsychological experiences occur. At the practical level this boils down to enhanced intuition and even a degree of thought reading which can be of immense value in the board room or across the negotiating table. I will therefore give you a brief survey, but a teacher would be required if you wanted to pursue this course.

Meditation is entered in three stages. From the experience of total relaxation or relaxation through music, painting, walking alone and so on, you can advance into *Jappa* or chanting to yourself. This takes the form of the continuous utterance of a single word or humming noise or a sound like *Allah-hoo* (as used in Sufism) or *oh-mm* (used by Hindus). The sound resonates in the brain and dulls the anxieties. The same effect has been achieved for centuries in churches all over the world by people taking part in hymns and prayers.

The next stage, *Dhyana* or concentration, is achieved when you create a new dominant thought by focusing on one spot or area. You stay silent, think of Jesus, look at the Cross, think of God, nature, the sun, the moon, a beautiful picture, green fields, a yellow spot on a darkened blackboard, a purple spot in the centre of your forehead. Concentrate on the point between your eyebrows, the third eye point. Such concentration does not actually use external agents such as sound or light.

The third stage is *Tappah*, true meditation, which means you bypass all blockages in the subconscious – you uplift yourself. This is the higher form. You push yourself beyond consciousness into a paraconscious state – the ethereal. This happens when you go into a trance. You go into a state where the block between conscious and subconscious is removed and they exchange information. You stop feeling your body, stop feeling all the aches and pains. It is like a total discharge of all the tension in different parts of the brain. It is a going beyond – bringing harmony in the whole body because the subconscious then functions as one with the conscious. You are at peace and all the organs that the subconscious brain controls get a certain amount of release from its attentions. High blood pressure and pulse rate come down, tolerance and threshold go up. Physical problems calm down.

Monks believe that if they do this they can achieve nirvana, the eternal peace. In itself meditation is entirely self-centred, though the results – serenity, improved intuition and mind control – may be put to good social or even business use. For most people, I recommend breathing and relaxation, as in the daily yoga exercises. The breathing technique helps mind control sufficiently for normal needs, but if time is available, and the desire to experience the superior powers is there, then by all means go ahead.

Chapter 7

Massage and Muscles

Massage is all to do with muscles. Most people think of a muscle as a piece of meat. After all, that's what you eat in a pork chop or a fillet steak. Actually it is an extremely complex organ filled with networks of nerves, fibres, blood vessels and attachments to tendons and ligaments. It is also a pump subsidiary to the heart and can pump blood throughout itself, a shaking you can often feel when you tax the muscle to its limit. This pumping action also generates heat, and is one of the main sources of heat in the body. When you rub your arms and legs to keep warm in the winter, you are not only increasing blood flow by the pumping action of the muscles, you are also using their inherent heat generation to warm you up through friction.

You can get some idea of the complexity of muscles by imagining the role of the leg muscles as you walk along a pavement, with all the tiny controls needed to maintain your gait and perhaps to step off the pavement to avoid a crowd of people. All the time you are able to maintain perfect balance, despite changes of height and weight distribution, especially if you have a bag of shopping. Just imagine what goes on in the muscles of a ballet dancer!

To achieve this degree of control the muscle can be in hundreds of independent sections, each playing its own part in the overall movement. Each of these has the capacity to go wrong. You can test this yourself by probing your calf or forearm muscles.

You may think they are relaxed as you sit in a comfortable chair, but as you push your thumb all over a muscle you are likely to find a few sore places. These are usually small pockets that have gone into spasm, like a tiny clenched fist, a minor case of the cramp which can be so painful when it covers the whole muscle. These spasms are stuck in that condition because the tightness has constricted the blood flow in that area. If you push on the sore place and gently massage it with your thumb or finger, the pain will dull, and if you do it every day for a few days it will go away altogether. The first time the pain is a bit unpleasant but, in the later stages of relaxation, massaging the soreness can be quite pleasurable because of the relief. You have then released the spasm and restored the flow of blood. Daily massage of the accessible muscles keeps you in trim and if you have a partner who can massage your spine, shoulders and neck you will feel in wonderful shape.

The value of massage

Historically, massage has long been practised as a means towards relaxation, muscle toning and hence health, and also as a therapy. Indeed it is instinctive. A little boy falls and hurts his knee. What does mother say? 'Rub it.' What do we do to gain the affection of domestic pets? Massage them. Hippocrates advised that massage, if strenuous, hardens the body, if gentle, relaxes; if much, it diminishes, if moderate, fills out. He therefore recommended massage when a feeble body has to be toned up, or one hardened or calloused has to be softened, or a harmful superfluity has to be dispersed, or a thin and infirm body has to be nourished. Massage was provided in the Greek healing temples, particularly for the first or crisis stage of an illness. In ancient Rome the emphasis was on maintenance of health. The wealthy would employ their own masseur, while the public would employ those who worked at the municipal baths. Massage also had a recuperative role for convalescents, especially those recovering from fever, and was used to bring relief to those suffering from prolonged headaches or a partially paralysed limb. In India in AD 600 Vagbhata included in his *Heart of Medicine* the advice that one should have a regular massage; it removes ageing, tiredness and wind, and improves the eyesight, vitality, sleep and complexion. He advised that particular attention should be given to the head, ears and feet but warned that massage is inappropriate for people who are full of phlegm, who have been purged or who have indigestion. He also recommended massage as a remedy for insanity. Though I add this somewhat light-heartedly, it does show that massage was regarded as having an effect on the mind. Traditionally in India people rubbed mustard oil all over their bodies and were massaged before taking a bath.

Once again, massage is an approach to treatment which has not only stood the test of time, but has the additional endorsement that it has developed independently, and been seen as an essential ingredient to health, by all traditional medicine. Those I have mentioned so far were concerned only with the direct muscular effect. The Chinese, however, went a stage further and related stimulation of the body surface to the acupuncture points they had already discovered, so combining the muscular benefits with the reflex features for toning up the internal organs. Thus developed acupressure in China and Shiatsu in Japan, both combining traditional massage with point pressures. In a specialist sense this was also independently developed in India, where stimulation of the marma points was used to relieve disabilities, pain and stiffness; I use this therapy today in stroke rehabilitation.

As I mentioned already, massage increases the blood circulation in the muscles. If you squeeze you expel the blood and, when you let go, more and fresh blood flows back in. There are other ways of doing this. In Thailand massage is taken very seriously, the main school being in one of the major temples in Bangkok, the Wat Po, and massage clinics are to be found all over the country. Here, massage is based on stretching ligaments and tendons, twisting joints, stretching muscles. It is another way of squeezing and releasing. The effect is similar. Masseurs often actually walk up and down people's spines. In Indonesia, in bomo massage, traditional healers used coins to scrape the muscles very deeply, bruising them. This activated the body and the bruising stimulated the immune system. In Turkey bears were trained to walk on people's backs. All this adds up to 2.5 billion people in Asia alone who believe in the therapeutic properties of massage. It has been a therapeutic system everywhere.

Muscles, massage and conventional medicine

So why does it lack popularity in the West? To answer that we have to look once more at conventional medicine, which has paid scant attention to muscles. According to conventional medicine muscles only contract, they do not expand. Even so doctors don't study the way they contract. For example the spine is supported by muscles. We stand erect because of an anti-gravitational force – something that pulls or pushes you up. Conventional medicine says muscles contract, although it might be more accurate to say they shrink. The muscle micro-fibres slide into each other. Now if muscles shrink, how do they create the anti-gravitational force that enables us to stand upright? There must be some muscles in the spine that actually extend upwards (expand). Perhaps some are like a long balloon – if you squeeze them in the middle (shrinkage), they get longer (expansion). If so, the middle of the muscle contracts, achieving elongation.

In between shrinking and expanding there is isometric contraction, when the muscles tighten without changing length, as in the case of the biceps when picking up a pail of water.

You can test muscle expansion with a simple experiment. Place your wrists together so that the lines at the bottom of the palms meet. Let your palms come together and, in a normal person, the tips of the fingers will also coincide. This is no surprise. Most people have two hands the same size. Now, choose a spot on the wall at shoulder height (whether sitting or standing). Stretch one arm out towards that spot, keeping your hand as relaxed as you can. Now concentrate very hard on that spot on the wall. Imagine the tips of your fingers reaching out towards that spot, getting nearer and nearer to it. Do this for about half a minute. Now, quickly put the lines at the bottom of your palms together, then the palms, then the tips of your fingers. Are your hands still the same length?

My conclusion is that muscles can expand as well as contract. Now, apply this principle to the spine. In the morning you are taller than in the evening by as much as 3.5 cm. During the day, body weight compresses the discs. If you tone up the muscles the effect is not so evident. The important point, however, is that the muscles in the spine shrink as they tire during the day and expand during the night as they recuperate (recovery time again). If you tone them up by massage, or add muscle bulk through nutrition and exercise they do not tire as much. Giving uncontrolled traction to stretch muscles beyond their natural elastic capacity is perhaps the worst thing one can do. Yet it is one of the standard treatments used in conventional medicine.

At one time I worked for a musicians' clinic where many artists who played the piano or a guitar lost power in their fingers at the peak of a performance. These artists usually took beta-blockers or anxiety-reducing pills, as such weird reactions were considered to be resulting from stress. The frog experiment in physiology I mentioned earlier (page 37) helped me to understand the condition of the musicians' fingers – the energy reserves in the muscles were being used up and the muscles needed time for recovery. A violinist came to me devastated that his left hand had seized up while playing a particularly brilliant passage. I began to massage his fingers and the muscles of the hand and arm and gave him resistance exercises to build up the muscle volume. Over a period of time the muscle bulk built up and so did the strength in the muscles. The artist stopped having cramps and he is now a well-known soloist, playing with leading symphony orchestras. What was happening here was that the recovery period of weak muscles was long and so the artist's fingers were incapacitated. Once the bulk and strength were built up, his fingers could work for a long time without getting fatigued.

The poor understanding of how muscles work has arisen because conventional doctors studied muscles *in vitro* (static or in laboratory conditions). They could not study muscles *in vivo*, the living or dynamic situation (because obviously it would be painful and unethical), so they missed out on some very vital clues about muscles. This is why conventional treatment of spinal disorders is so poor and whole new professions, such as osteopathy and chiropractic, have emerged to fill the gap.

Using massage as a treatment

Backache

When I am treating or trying to prevent backaches I try to make the muscles extend the spine, with the help of massage and spinal exercises. To me the spine is one entity and I treat it as such. All nerves emerge from the spine and go into different parts of the body, so the spine is very important. I massage not only the muscles of the spine, but also the tendons at the ends of the muscles, because the tendons can be sore and taut if the muscles are tight. Tendons are tough and have poor blood supply. That is why they are white in colour and hard. So the injuries that take place in tendons are more difficult to cure than muscle injuries, where there is a good blood supply. There are small blood vessels on the outside of the tendons and by massaging them, through friction, I try to improve what circulation there is.

The neck

The massage of the neck is very essential. If you look at the anatomy of the neck (see opposite) you will see that the vertebrae have canals on both sides. Through this pair of vertebral canals pass the vertebral arteries, the most vital blood vessels in the body. These arteries supply blood to the subconscious part of the brain (as opposed to the carotid arteries on the front part of the neck which predominantly supply blood to the cortex or conscious part of the brain). The subconscious brain includes the vital centres (respiratory, cardiovascular), cranial nerve centres, appetite centre, gait, posture, balance centres, the pituitary (master hormonal gland controlling thyroid, adrenalin, stress, reproductive hormones), emotional centres, sleep centres etc. Thus vertebral arteries control most of our subconscious functions. If the blood flow through them is good the feeling of wellbeing is positive. Spasms of neck muscles or disalignment of the vertebrae of the neck can impair blood flow through the vertebral arteries and thus create grounds for fatigue, headaches, dizziness, malaise, poor hormonal functions, insomnia, etc.

I have studied the role of vertebral arteries for over 17 years and have come to the conclusion that their normal function is vital to wellbeing and prevention of a whole range of diseases. I therefore give a lot of emphasis on neck massage.

Muscular cramps and stiffness

There are a few other muscular conditions that cry out for massage. The whole body is in a very strange situation if the muscles are tight due to tension or stress. You have created a block in the circulatory system, which is the most important system. When you massage muscles, especially tight muscles, you release the spasms and hence the resistance to blood flow. Head massage plays an important role in stress management. Coconut oil or similar oils can be massaged into the scalp. In Indian systems of massage, head massage always plays an important part. The scalp is toned up with gentle movement of the fingers. This improves blood flow to the brain as most of the blood from it drains out into the veins in the scalp region.

An extreme case of muscle spasm is **cramp**. Muscles go into a cramp when there is a lack of calcium and lack of blood flow. It is a chemical reaction and a whole group of

The anatomy of the neck

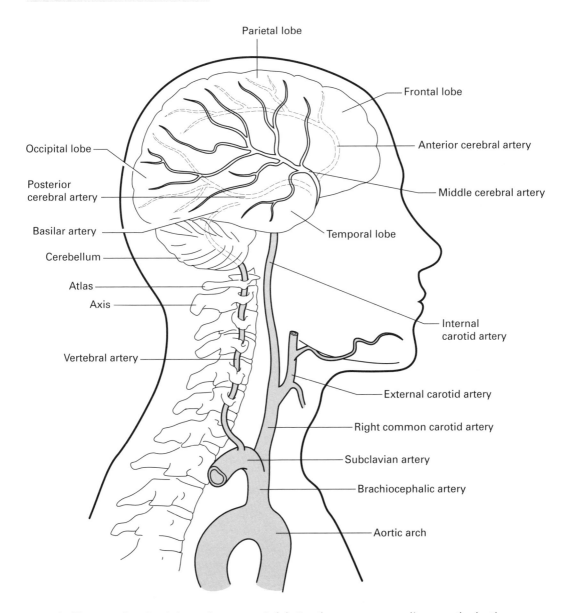

Parietal lobe

Frontal lobe

Occipital lobe

Anterior cerebral artery

Posterior
cerebral artery

Middle cerebral artery

Basilar artery

Temporal lobe

Cerebellum

Atlas

Axis

Internal
carotid artery

Vertebral artery

External carotid artery

Right common carotid artery

Subclavian artery

Brachiocephalic artery

Aortic arch

muscle fibres are involved. It can be very painful. Gentle massage can disperse the lactic acid and toxins, recover the circulation and relieve the cramp. Writer's cramp is quite common in people who write a lot. The index fingers can straighten up involuntarily and cannot bend again for a period of time (the recovery period). Those who constantly use keyboards and work very fast face similar problems. Many of these injuries or abnormal hand phenomena are classified now as repetitive strain injury (RSI). I now advise those who do this type of job (quick movements over a prolonged period) to rest their hands and massage the strained muscles to free them from accumulated lactic acid. Lactic acid is a by-product of glucose metabolism. Normally when oxygen comes into contact with glucose they combine into carbon dioxide and water, which have no effect on the muscles. If, however, the supply of oxygen is reduced, or the muscles are demanding more oxygen than can be supplied, the glucose gets converted into lactic acid, an intermediate product. Only when you are able to supply more oxygen does the lactic acid get converted into carbon dioxide and water.

Stiffness is another condition caused by a build-up of lactic acid. Many joggers will be familiar with the problem of stiffness in the calves when they first take up the exercise, or if they restart it after a longish rest. After a few days of painful jogging, however, the stiffness goes and does not return. This phenomenon occurs because when exercising for the first time or after a break the muscles are not fit. The strain on the muscles causes an accumulation of lactic acid, which can be dispersed by massage. With greater muscle bulk the same activity can be performed without strain. But you have to keep it up. When people give up sport their muscles atrophy and they get a lot of cramps as a result of shrinkage of the muscles.

As I mentioned earlier, Greek and Indian massage was mainly soothing and squeezing. My massage is much deeper, finding sore spots. Massage should be deep, because as soon as you press the muscles, especially the sore areas, a certain amount of spasm or tenseness is induced. It is a guarding effect to prevent pain but it can prevent the therapeutic effect of massage. Massage can't be just superficial treatment – to achieve a therapeutic effect you have to press the muscles fairly deeply. The idea is to squeeze the muscles so that, as you remove the pressure, they expand and draw in blood. Basically you are seeking to get more oxygen and blood into the muscles. Occasionally, weaker blood vessels might bruise. This is natural and is a temporary effect which affects only the weaker blood vessels, not the healthy ones. If they bruise, new blood vessels are formed. It is not a problem.

Healing

Never forget that you are not just massaging, you are touching, and this initiates a healing process of its own. Don't underestimate the power of healing through the hands. It has been well documented in history back to Jesus Christ and beyond. It is instinctive for a mother to use her healing powers by placing a hand on her baby when it is sick. During my medical course at university I was taught to focus my mind through my hands to achieve healing and I still practise this, at least as an adjunct, in all my healing work. One member of my staff at the Integrated Medical Centre is a healer and has spent his life doing nothing else, often with astounding results. Most people who reject healing do so because they can't fathom how it works. I have to admit neither can I. One of the great strengths of traditional and now integrated medicine is the ability to accept processes that work, even if they cannot be explained scientifically. Acupuncture is perhaps the outstanding example of this.

Maybe I can give sceptics some help in appreciating healing by explaining it this far. A TV remote controller sends out a beam of heat (scientists call it infra-red). The beam is coded to select different channels. Is it too much to expect that the heat emanating from the body or from the healer's hands is also coded, allowing the healer to sense a great deal about the patient's state of health, and allowing the patient to accept power or instructions from the healer to stimulate the physis? In other words the patient does the healing with the help and stimulation of the healer. So massage should include a high degree of sensitivity to the condition of the patient and the results to be achieved.

How to massage

A critical question is, can you do it yourself? The answer is not only 'Yes', but 'You should'. You can keep your legs, arms and shoulders in trim, using thumb or finger pressure to look for sore spots (it's easier for you to find them than for anyone else). Press down a line of points on each side of the bones and down the middle of the muscles. You'll soon find them. Then a gentle rotary action or just still pressure can usually clear the soreness quite quickly. You can take your calf and forearm muscles by the handful and squeeze and release them. To keep good circulation in the limbs this way is highly beneficial.

An even better way is to do it is as a partnership. Take it in turns to treat your partner. Run up the muscles in the limbs and buttocks. Use finger or thumb pressure to run up either side of the spine, digging, not too roughly, into the cavities between the sides of the vertebrae. Using the palms of your hands you can even put much of your weight directly on the vertebrae all the way up, like a Turkish bear. Shoulders and neck are particularly important. Dig your thumbs into the muscles below and above the shoulder blades and up each side of the neck. Don't forget the scalp. Follow this routine for 10–20 minutes each, every night before you go to bed, and you will be amazed how it will improve your sleep and your performance.

Just a few warnings. Keep the room warm and well ventilated. Work at a comfortable height on a firm bed or mat. Don't wear jewellery, wrist watches or anything that could scratch the skin. That goes for fingernails too. Keep them smooth and as short as you can. Warm up your hands first. Pour the oil (aromatic oils are best) on to your hands, not on to your partner. Use your whole body action and focus on what you are trying to achieve. That means keeping talking to a minimum. Don't do it straight after a meal. Avoid obvious weak areas, varicose veins, the abdomen of a pregnant woman, injuries, infections or fractures of bony areas. Play relaxing music, but not music that is heavily rhythmic.

Chapter 8

INDIVIDUALITY

CONSTITUTION AND TEMPERAMENT

Your constitution is your physical and mental make-up – what you were born with. You might have a strong constitution, meaning you are essentially healthy. Someone with a weak constitution might be constantly ill. Temperament, on the other hand, is your manner of thinking, behaving or reacting. You might have an even, a nervous or a fiery temperament, but this can be both controlled and modified; it is something you acquire and it depends upon what you eat, what your character is, how you indulge things and so on. Medically speaking the important word is 'reacting', for someone with an even temperament may react evenly to stress, while the nervous person may fall ill under the same pressure. We are all individuals.

Some people can eat a lot of food and still remain thin, whereas others may put on weight with even small amounts of food. Some sleep better, get less exhausted, are cheerful and generally enjoy life more than others. The thing that makes one type of person different from another is the constitution. It is a very important part of our life and yet medical science has not been able to study it. If it were studied in depth and the knowledge applied to the findings of modern physiology, conventional doctors would have a better chance of understanding the human body and mind. This would improve our knowledge of medicine which, according to the great physician Avicenna, is a science by which we learn the various states of the human body in health and sickness, and the means by which health is likely to be lost and, when lost, how it is likely to be restored.

So both constitution and temperament affect your health, and may even affect whether you are regarded as healthy or not. A rattle in a ten-year-old Ford might be acceptable, but not in a ten-year-old Rolls Royce. A melancholic person could, because of his negative nature, live close to the borderline of sickness but not be ill, while an energetic, enthusiastic person displaying the same symptoms and the same results when his temperature and blood pressure are checked (thus registering as 'not sick') might in fact be quite seriously ill because he had drifted so far from his constitutional norm. Conventional science no longer takes this individual variation into account, apart from in certain specialised areas such as blood group, or gender – i.e. those variations that can be established scientifically – whereas it is fundamental to all traditional medicine. A careless cook will put an egg in boiling water for a few minutes and produce a variety of runny or hard-boiled eggs. The good cook will judge the size, weight and shape of the egg, the room temperature and the heat of the stove, and will adjust the cooking time accordingly. That cook will achieve much greater consistency in his boiled eggs. So the physician who correctly judges the constitution and temperament of patients will take better care of their health.

Centuries ago physicians realised that people differed in certain fundamental ways, and that these differences affected their response to disease and to treatment. Long ago they tried to classify these differences by referring to observable effects on the body under different conditions. For example, if a person behaved and appeared as if he were being subjected to warmth or heat, if he was energetic and socially active, they referred to his condition as being 'hot'. This did not mean his temperature was any different from anyone else, it was only symbolic. If he was huddled up in a corner he was 'cold'. Thus temperamental variations were referred to as hot, cold, dry and moist, to indicate how a person appeared.

Humours

Hippocrates put forward the theory that the body contained four fluids, which he called 'humours', defined as blood, phlegm, yellow bile (choler) and black bile. Avicenna later isolated these as being derived in digestion, the blood humour being, as he put it, hot and moist and carrying the superior nutrients to heart and cells. It is dominant in spring, in childhood, and in the air. The phlegm humour, cold and moist, is converted by digestion into mucus, saliva, and gastric and intestinal fluids. It is dominant in summer, youth and in fire. The yellow or bilious humour, hot and dry, or 'normal' bile, was formed from the residue in the liver and used for digestion in the duodenum. It is dominant in autumn, maturity and in the earth. The residual black bile affected spleen, blood and phlegm. It is dominant in winter, old age and in water. At every stage abnormalities resulted in the production of toxins which had to be eliminated. An excess or dominance of a particular humour, however, could be the constitutional norm.

The concept of 'humour' is still used today: even the most up-to-date dictionary will tell you that humour is a body fluid such as blood, lymph or bile, the aqueous and vitreous humours are fluids in the eye, and when we talk of a child of sullen humour or say we are 'in no humour to argue' or 'out of humour', we are still referring to constitution and temperament.

That the Hippocratic theory of humours has stood the test of time for 2,500 years may not be the most surprising aspect of this. What is astounding, as I mentioned in Chapter 2, is that the Indians and the Chinese developed theories and categories of constitution and temperament completely independently from the Greeks and from each other and yet these theories were remarkably similar. In all traditions it was recognised that all the humours existed in everyone, but it was the dominance of one that determined a person's personality and his or her health needs. Furthermore, personality (temperament) varied with age, so these needs were constantly changing.

For example, a fever in an elderly person is treated quite differently from a fever in a child because of their temperaments. It is therefore surprising to find herbal encyclopaedias listing herbs suitable for treating a fever without reference to age or any other characteristic of temperament. One might say this is a useful test of the reliability of the encyclopaedia. A person's temperament is revealed in his appearance. A ruddy complexion indicates a dominance of the blood humour, a pinkish skin shows a balanced temperament, and black or yellow tones in the skin can indicate the dominance of other humours. If appearance is at variance with the person's normal temperament it can be a signpost to disease, which the traditional practitioner will be quick to notice.

Until the beginning of the nineteenth century even conventional medicine accepted the four types of human beings. Hanhemann, the father of homoeopathy, spoke of the constitution some 200 years ago and formulated his famous constitutional remedies. Various philosophers or scientists attempted to make their own classification. For example Jung (1923) divided people into Extroverts and Introverts. Pavlov, the great Russian physiologist, divided people into Lively, Impetuous, Calm and Weak. It is the great weakness in 'scientific' assessments of drugs or bodily reactions to external agents today that the statistics are based on groups of people who are assumed to be equal. Such tests do not take into account the different constitutions within the groups. All such so-called scientific analysis is of questionable value.

A particular example of this is to be found in the variations of people's sensitivity to the environment. Some people are more sensitive than others to radiation from TV screens, mobile phones or power cables. For example I can feel pressure in my sternum when I pass through a security gate at the airport. I believe this is rare. Some, probably most, people can take any amount of such radiation, but for a few people it makes them ill. It's a question of threshold. The result is that when medical science studies the effect of such radiation on the human body, as far as I can gather they take the statistical average of all people exposed to such radiation and come up with the conclusion that there is no convincing evidence that such radiation is harmful. I suspect that if they surveyed those who are sensitive, who have experienced ill effects, they would come up with a very different conclusion.

AGE

In no aspect are the different appearances and conflicting needs of different temperaments clearer than in variations of age. Shakespeare observed there were seven ages of man: the infant, the whining schoolboy, the lover, the soldier, the justice, the retired gentleman (in lean and slippered pantaloon) and second childhood. Such were his extraordinary powers of observation that he correctly described the temperaments of each age, the lover being melancholic, the soldier sanguine, the old judge phlegmatic, and so on. Shakespeare would have had the apothecary prescribe differently for each.

Avicenna defined four ages – childhood, youth, maturity and old age – as being predominantly sanguine, choleric, melancholic and phlegmatic, thus departing somewhat from Shakespeare, possibly by failing to take into account the propensity of young people to fall in love, which alters their temperament, usually temporarily. (One might ask, however, that if love results in such a departure from the temperamental norm is it indeed, as Shakespeare so often said, a sickness?)

Observation shows that age does play an important part in health and reveals differences in predisposition to disease. The growth period during youth is positive, with more assimilation than dissimilation. More cells are built up than destroyed. Then there comes a status quo, a plateau from, say, the age of 25 to 60, when there is no growth and no loss of cells or tissue. What you use you replenish. After that comes a stage when you build less and lose more. You lose fat, hair, teeth, eyesight and hearing. The arteries become more restricted and the heart is not so strong. An integrated medical practitioner will be sensitive to differences every seven years of life, though in broad terms, he recognises, unlike Shakespeare, five ages of man.

Childhood and adolescence

Up to the age of seven, while the immune system is developing, a child is most vulnerable to disease and needs the greatest care. Infant mortality worldwide is a major loss to parents and to the population. A child that passes the age of seven has a good chance of reaching middle age.

The teenage years are a period of stubbornness and revolt against childhood teaching, creating bad habits and practices which may become permanent. For a physician, teenagers can be a nightmare (and the elderly are the next worst). I have even declined to treat teenagers' allergies, asthma and eczema, because these conditions are diet-related and to treat them would be impossible. The children at that age have absolutely no discipline. I tell the parents we will have to wait till they grow up. I always try and impress on parents to bring their children in before they are teenagers so they can be treated. I am aware, of course, that the teenagers do not suffer much. It is a generally healthy time of life, but I like to make sure they enter the teenage years as healthy as I can make them. Diseases like anorexia, acne, manic-depressive disorders etc in teenagers are particularly difficult to treat because they are related to age, diet and psychological factors. It is a treble whammy.

Adulthood

The 20s and 30s are a period when misuse of the body can usually be handled by the youthful sanogenetic powers, leading to a person taking them for granted after their powers decline. By this time parental influence has also declined, and there are major difficulties in convincing youths that the time has come to settle down from their teenage excesses and create a lifestyle that will keep them healthy indefinitely. However, people in this age bracket are mature and are often health conscious. Certain diseases such as multiple sclerosis, schizophrenia, chronic fatigue syndrome, late asthma (different from childhood asthma) tend to develop between twenty and forty.

Middle age

People have to be very careful between the ages of 40 and 60. Statistically, this is a dangerous period. The arteries have begun to harden and changes in hormones take place. This is the period in life when all the intemperance of youth comes home to roost in the form of heart attacks, cancer, cirrhosis, gout, succumbing to stress, chronic fatigue due to lack of muscular care, digestive disorders – you name it. This age is characterised by more frequent visits to the doctor for check-ups or because of sickness and is the time when people get loaded up with prescription drugs. In April 1998 the *Journal of the American Medical Association* (Vol 279, no 15) estimated that adverse reactions to prescription drugs are killing about 106,000 Americans each year. It is to be expected that the 40–60 age group is the one that suffers most in this respect. It is a time when the Lifestyle Programme becomes a life-saver. In a sense this book targets people aged 40–60, though if people can become adjusted to a healthy lifestyle before that they will have done themselves a terrific service.

Integrated medicine can do much to mitigate the problems associated with this period of life, such as the menopause and declining energy levels. I recommend a high-protein diet during the **menopause**. Coffee, excess salt, smoking, alcohol and drugs should be avoided as they excite the nervous system. Yoga is very beneficial because it improves the circulation, boosts energy levels and relaxes the mind. A weekly massage, especially of the neck and shoulders, helps to reduce fatigue. Herbal remedies that mimic oestrogen are useful: try two capsules of freeze-dried aloe vera once a day, or 1 teaspoon of Shatavari powder mixed with half a teaspoon of kolonji oil and a little honey, once a day. Mexican yam capsules or extract help to alleviate hot flushes. You should combine this with vitamin supplements containing Vitamins B1 and B6, magnesium and selenium.

To boost **energy levels in middle age**, I recommend regular deep tissue massages, regular walks in the fresh air and supplements such as Vitamin B complex with magnesium (150 mg tablets once a day) or one teaspoon of Ashwagandha (Indian ginseng) with honey once a day.

People who pass the age of 60 have a good chance of reaching 80. In general these are folks who have led a reasonable lifestyle, have practised moderation and diversity in their diet and exercise, have avoided overindulgence in smoking and alcohol, and have kept clear of drugs, both illicit and prescribed.

Old age

Old age presents its own particular chronic problems, which are often not life-threatening, only uncomfortable and, surprisingly, often reversible. Much of old age is in the mind. Some people, on reaching a critical age, are surprised to find nothing has changed and they don't feel old until the age of 80 or more. Others start to grow old at 50. The fact is if you allow yourself to grow old you will. I have known people retire and then drop dead the following next week, or couples where when one dies and the other loses the will to live. Elderly people who are neglected or cast aside soon die. When I was working with the Namdhari Sikhs in India we used to pick up elderly dying people from the streets and house them in a building with good care and pleasant surroundings. We gave them something to live for and many lived for another ten years. The prescription is often no more than tender loving care and an incentive.

On the other hand I have known chief executives who retired and took up another job, then another, and continued to keep their minds active for years. The number of elderly is growing at least in part because of the variety of activities available to them. Of course improved health care for the elderly is also a big contributor. Treating the elderly is an art in itself. They are often like children, in that they don't speak their minds. If they are unhappy they keep it to themselves. It is often difficult to dig out the real problem.

People in non-Western societies seem to know when their time has come. In the remote Himalayas and among the Inuit, old people living on their own simply get up and go out and die. But choosing to give up on life is different. It's a choice. If you give up you give in. If you keep yourself active and take all the precautionary (lifestyle) measures, you should be able to go on indefinitely. If you are not working your eating habits should change and your general lifestyle should also change accordingly.

The encouraging thing about growing old is that you are at the height of experience, knowledge and wisdom and you approach true maturity. Maturity occurs when you have collected enough experience to be able to know the laws of nature, to know how things are in nature, to be able to say from experience that you know about family values, life as it goes, the weather. You have more fixed views that come from experience. Your decisions become firmer, less flexible. When you make a decision you know it is correct and you can stick by it. Prior to that you might listen to other people's advice, dither, be messy-minded, but ultimately, if the decision is your own, that is a strong sign of maturity. (One might say traditional medicine is mature, though conventional medicine has not reached that stage.)

True maturity is a later stage, as a generality applying to the over-60s. It is a stage when you can acquire more knowledge and information for your own interest, but you have achieved what you set out to do in life. A child learns not to touch hot things, put its fingers in an electrical socket, or go out on a balcony in case it falls. The child learns from experience. These experiences through life – the teenage years, menstruation, first sexual contact, having a baby, the skills you acquire – all these things add up to a mature stage. But at around 60 you don't acquire new skills, you live on your experience. For the purpose of knowledge you still want to know, but you don't use it as part of your experience. You don't bring in new changes. For example, if you tell a 60-year-old who has drunk alcohol regularly to give it up he says 'I have done this all my life'. He won't change. Indeed, the main problem with old people is their habits. It is very difficult to get them to do something different. If you start them on exercises, they might do it for a few days but then stop.

Age, however, can determine health, and many of the problems of ill health in the elderly are not only preventable but reversible. Sinus disorders, constipation, failing eyesight, chronic fatigue, insomnia, loss of short-term memory and osteoarthritis are all preventable and reversible. In particular, osteoarthritis is curable (see page 169 for details of treatment). So take care, keep the mind active, walk and work in the garden, have light dinners, normal lunches and drink alcohol – always in moderation. To some all this comes naturally, but do it and you will enjoy your old age just like you did the rest of your life. Do not forget to pray and leave time for spiritual development.

Wisdom

My deep regret is that the wisdom of old age is no longer being passed on. Most children are leaving home at twenty-one or earlier and live their own lives. In this way, the extended family system has collapsed with grandparents no longer teaching their grandchildren the values of life and mothers and grandmothers no longer teaching their daughters and daughters-in-law the values of child care. When stressed you go to a counsellor for help instead of your parents or family and school teachers are taking up the role of moulding habits and characters. The old knowledge is not being passed on and a lot has passed away and has been lost forever. Many of the old sayings had deep philosophical connotations but today they are regarded as superstition or just fables.

Chapter 9

THE MIND

There is another reason why individuals differ from each other in their state of health and their reaction to treatment and that is because they can think – and they think differently. Now in conventional medicine this does not matter much because, except in the certain specialised areas, physiology does not study the link between the mind and the body. Let us, however, examine this link and see how much it does matter.

THE MIND-BODY LINK

You have an erotic thought. What happens? There is a physical effect and the only cause that can be found is the original thought. The conscious brain has not activated any muscles or made any physical alteration to the body. All it has done is activate the subconscious mind that controls the involuntary nervous system and the hormonal system. There is a mind–body link. But what caused the thought? It could have been a word, or catching someone's eye. So the thought could have had a physical origin, passing through the body, via the ear or the eye, to the mind. It is therefore a two-way link.

The human brain has two different sides: one makes you active, the other slows you down. We call it manic and depressive. You can see this in the moods you experience: 'I feel low' or 'I feel good'. The two sides of the brain are in conflict, it is a split in personality. Conflict is at the root of most stress. A lot of diseases are caused by dilemmas, having to decide between two conflicting aims; it's the most stressful thing a human being can face. In the animal kingdom, if you put a donkey between two haystacks, such is its lack of intelligence that it will die of starvation rather than decide which to eat from. The other human menace is deadlines. The nervous system follows a certain rhythm and pattern. When you hurry it up you become stressed because the mind has its own cyclical pattern. You may be able to complete the work in a certain period but the moment you create a deadline you create stress. Deadlines, dilemmas and human relationships are the three major causes of stress. They are an outside influence on the brain. Internal influences are caused by pain, disease, discomfort, insomnia, indigestion which in themselves are very stressful.

How does the body affect the mind?

Much has been written about psychosomatic disease and the power of the mind in controlling physical turmoil in the body. Some people have gone overboard and are obsessed with the idea of 'mind over matter'. You can cure anything, including cancer, using your mind – so they say. This, I feel, is a Utopian idea, a tall order. However, physical factors such as the supply of blood to the brain can have an effect on the functioning of the mind. When the brain receives a good blood supply, you feel well. The brain cells are very susceptible to glucose fluctuations. For example, someone with hypoglycaemia, (low blood sugar), gets jittery and panicky with a nervous sinking feeling; the brain is dull; thinking and vision become blurred. Recently the mapping of the brain has shown that lack of oxygen and glucose to different parts of the brain can cause various diseases. So the brain has to be looked after physically. The body is the temple in which the mind thrives. You can't have a healthy mind without a healthy body. So let's see what else can affect the brain.

Excess sugar can make children hyperactive. Excess coffee can make people very irritable and agitated. Substance abuse affects the brain, as do many food additives. For example MSG makes people nervous; excessive salt makes people tense. Therefore there are food substances (including recreational drugs and alcohol) that alter the mind, which is the functional manifestation of the brain.

It is important to know that general physiological problems can affect the mind. For example, a pain in the left side of the chest causes panic, because everyone thinks it is their heart (though it might not be – it could be neurological pain from the back, or pleurisy, or muscular spasm). Diabetes, cancer and chronic ailments alter the way you think because you so often worry about the consequences of the disease. Shakespeare once said, 'There never was philosopher that could endure the toothache'. He was right, toothache can be the cause of great irritability. Problems such as impotence or premenstrual syndrome can cause psychological disturbance. With premenstrual syndrome, women get mood changes just before their periods. Hormonal imbalance can have a psychological effect. Depression can be due to lack of vitamins and minerals. Conditions such as chronic constipation can make you tired. If you sweat excessively it can make you tired, irritable and depressed. This is because of electrolyte loss which causes nervous tissues to malfunction. An over-active thyroid can make you crazy, make you want to kill. In general, if the pathogenetic powers are too strong, if stress is too great or you haven't slept for so many nights, then the mind is seriously affected. You break down, you have obsessions, persecutions, hallucinations, while the sanogenetic powers strive to keep a balance.

On the other hand the body's influence on the mind can be used positively. If you are anxious and having panic attacks you can stop them by carrying out certain breathing exercises. High blood pressure can be controlled by relaxation or meditation techniques. These dilate the blood vessels and slow down the heart rate so that the blood pressure comes down – especially in the early stages of the condition when the blood pressure level is variable. Hiccups, initiated in the diaphragm, are a reflex action by the brain transmitted through the involuntary nervous system. It is a mind-generated effect which can be cured by drinking water or holding your breath.

Mind control

Conversely, the mind can control the actual physiology of the body. With willpower you can control breathing in asthma attacks, or avoid scratching the itchy skin in eczema. When tackling addictions you have to build up willpower in order to overcome physical cravings. In controlling pain you can build up your threshold by being positive. With life-threatening diseases such as cancer, unless you have a positive psychic approach, treatment is difficult because, particularly in cancer, the negative forces are strong – you think you are going to die, or you think it is the end of life. These are very powerful feelings but you have to counteract them. If you neutralise these feelings it makes a difference to the progression of the cancer, it slows it down. You can control feelings through meditation. Mind control can be so strong that people can actually walk over red hot charcoal without feeling any discomfort or suffering any damage to the feet. You can see this very often in the Hindu practices in India and Singapore. I even knew of an Irish lady who had learned to do it.

You see, the mind lays down priorities. Pain follows the law of dominance. Suppose you have toothache, right shoulder degeneration, a kidney stone, migraine and glaucoma – all at once, and all painful conditions. The pain of glaucoma will suppress everything else. You won't feel any other pain. But soon as the glaucoma is successfully treated you begin to feel the migraine. When that is cured the toothache takes over. The whole body cannot hurt at the same time. So it is with meditation or higher forms of mind control. They can dominate and you won't even feel hot coals under your feet. Plastic surgeons use this principle successfully. They will do a facelift, nose job and liposuction at the same time. All three areas will hurt and as a result you may not feel much pain as the brain cannot differentiate between them.

If someone is depressed or anxious you make them angry. It cures them every time. The hormones induced by anger are far more powerful than anything causing depression. If you tickle someone physically they laugh. The response has gone via the brain. More than that, the laughter makes other people laugh. You can see this clearly in the theatre – everyone laughs at all the jokes, whether they think they are funny or not, because other people's laughter makes them laugh. It is part of the psychic system, another system not taught in conventional medicine, which covers the whole of our communication with other people. It is not only a mind–body reaction, it is a mind–other-people's-bodies reaction. This is why death of an important personality, like Mahatma Gandhi, can cause mass psychosis and hysteria.

It follows from this that the beliefs and behaviour of physicians strongly influence the internal healing powers of the patients. If the patient has faith in the doctor it is a huge help, though I say this with reservations. Faith is not usually 'blind' but is built on certain foundations. Human beings are naturally suspicious, so they check out their physician. How many people visit this doctor? How busy is he and how well qualified? If a disease is purely psychological, then the doctor's beliefs and behaviour will make a difference; if not, there will be no difference. But then again, so many diseases are multifactorial that the doctor's own psyche is almost bound to play some part. We used to call it bedside manner. All this should be taught in general medicine.

Although we classify all nervous control into conscious and subconscious, there is another category in between these. Most habits can be conscious as well as subconscious. Gait, posture, speech, writing, swimming, breathing, swallowing, urination and so on, are controlled by both types of mind. When one learns a skill such as writing, swimming, walking, talking, one uses the voluntary mind, but after it is learnt it becomes under the control of the subconscious. You learn to write A, B, C, D; then you write words like apple, bird, cow, duck and after that you write sentences automatically and the hands move simultaneously with your thoughts. Learning to ride a bicycle is another typical example of how the conscious function is converted into subconscious and balance becomes far better as a result.

Conversely, there are some functions – the analysis of vision, sound, light, smell, memory, decision-making, emotions – that appear instinctive but can be controlled. For example, if there is grief you have it whether you want it or not. It's there. The emotion automatically follows the circumstance. But once it is there you may be able to control it, just as you can control breathing and sleep. Gait and posture are automatic but controllable. You can walk faster or slower, though the actual contraction of muscles or groups of muscles is involuntary.

You can train yourself to control just about anything. People have been able to sublimate their sexual energy and become more creative, utilising the sexual desire, a subconscious instinct, and diverting it to a different conscious activity. Buddhist monks only have thin bed-sheets and sleep on ice. Yet they generate so much body heat by mentally controlling it that they feel hot even lying down on snow. It is a form of adaptation. To control the mind to this extent, however, you have to train yourself. That is another aspect of medicine which is not taught to medical students.

Adaptation

Adaptation is as much a sign of life as reproduction, digestion, response to external stimuli and so on. Evolution took place because of constant adaptation to the changing environment. Human beings as part of the living world also constantly adapt themselves. Threshold and adaptation are interlinked. If you adapt, your threshold changes. You can take more of what you have adapted to. We have adapted to modern living. On average today we only sleep six hours instead of the traditional eight. We live longer. We have become used to canned products containing as many as ten potentially harmful chemicals.

If a man used to living near the sea were taken to live at 4,000 m, where the oxygen level is low, his body would be forced to adapt to the rarefied air or else he would not be able to survive. He would have all the symptoms of altitude sickness – headache, nausea, irregular breathing pattern, feeling disorientated, and so on. But as time went by his body's reserve mechanism would gear up the adaptation process. Within a few days the bone marrow would produce more red blood cells, his thirst and his appetite would increase and his breathing would become deeper. All these changes would take place due to adaptogenic forces, part of the sanogenetic forces in the body.

This is happening to us every day in so many ways that we are not aware of it. We adapt to a prolonged period of sunshine: our skin goes dark. We go away on business and adapt to hotel life. We fly halfway round the world and within a day or two have adapted to the new time. Our partner becomes sick and immediately we adapt to the new household regimen. At a physiological level we adapt to changes in our environment. Pollution increases and most of us adapt to it and don't get sick. There are traces of pesticides on our vegetables and fruit. Provided this does not exceed our tolerance level we may get symptoms such as fatigue or nausea at first but then we adapt to it. Recent studies have shown signs of a decline of asthma in children in the UK. It is possible that this is in part due to adaptation to pollution allergens.

Adaptation is going on inside us all the time. Consider homeostasis, the maintenance of body constants. The acid/alkali balance (the pH value) in the blood remains constant, even if you drink a litre of citrus juice (acid) or a cup of Angostura bitters (alkali). If the blood becomes more alkaline for some reason you retain carbon dioxide and turn it into carbonic acid, which neutralises the alkali. The optimum number of blood cells is maintained despite all outside influences, even a wound and loss of blood. The body temperature is constant in spite of the weather. It's a miraculous balancing act in view of the phenomenal changes taking place in the internal and external environment, changes caused by what you eat and drink and any vigorous exercise you might take. No engineer could design such perfect adaptation; it is the most amazing thing we have inherited from nature.

The adaptation process can work against us too. If we are put on blood pressure pills for a prolonged period our bodies adapt to the drugs and they become less effective. A physician will keep a close check on this and there can be two results: one physician may say the disease is getting worse and increase the dose; another will say you are adapting to the drug and change it. The same principles apply to supplements. Your body will adapt to a regular dose, which will lose its efficacy, just like the blood pressure pills. So long as you absorb a particular vitamin or mineral from a varied intake of vegetables you can keep the process up indefinitely. But take it every day in the form of the same pill and before long that pill will be going straight through your system and the nutrients will not be adequately absorbed. Your body will have adapted to it. So the old science-fiction idea of men existing permanently on pills could never work.

On the whole, however, adaptation is to be encouraged, and there are herbal adaptogens which help in this. One is ginseng or Ashwagandha, the Indian variety. It helps in better utilisation of oxygen in cells. It helps to transport oxygen though the cell walls. This helps to produce more energy in the tissues. The metabolic rate also increases in the tissues and therefore all the functions of the body are carried out at an increased pace. This facilitates adaptation. Ginseng is one of nature's natural life supporters. It gives the body extra energy, prevents plaque formation in arteries (arteriosclerosis), increases tissue repair (in case of trauma, bruises or cuts), improves parts of the immune system, improves blood circulation and stimulates the nervous system, thus increasing memory and brain power.

Ginseng, whether Siberian, Korean or Indian counterparts, is a root of rhizoma, similar to the ginger family. Its active ingredients have long been used in traditional medicine, for a variety of purposes, from improving sexual function to curing low blood pressure and chronic ailments like rheumatoid arthritis. The Soviets at one time tried Siberian ginseng to cure stomach ulcers, impotence, chronic fatigue, arthritis and depression. There were some isolated reports of success in these treatments.

In fact the Russians were probably the first to study adaptation in depth scientifically. Pavlov was one of the greatest physiologists the world has ever known. He lived between 1849 and 1935. He discovered what he called 'Conditional reflex'. 'Conditioning' is another way of describing adaptation. The essence of the conditional reflex was shown in experiments on dogs. The acid secretion in the stomachs of dogs was studied under different conditions. A bell or flashing light warned the dogs that they were about to be fed, so they associated these signals with food. After many trial runs these signals produced large amounts of acid in the stomach even before food was eaten.

Our whole life is dominated by these subconscious conditional reflexes. Around lunch time the stomach acids build up and hunger, irritability and impatience build up quite uncontrollably. We are conditioned to a particular time, say 1 p.m., as lunch time. There are more complex conditional reflexes than this simple type. At the beginning of summer when the pollen count in the air begins to rise, hay fever sufferers begin to get very alarmed and uncomfortable as they know the various symptoms like running nose, itchy eyes, sneezing and lethargy all too well from previous years. Hypochondriacs have the most extreme of all conditional reflexes. A headache is interpreted as a sign of brain tumour, a stomach cramp as a bursting of the appendix and a cough is taken as lung cancer or pneumonia. These people actually behave as if they have these ailments. Think how difficult it is for doctors to differentiate between the patient who is trying not to make a fuss and another who is exaggerating or seeking attention (temperament again). This is an important reason why a doctor's powers of examination and on-the-spot diagnosis have to rise above patients' own assessment of their condition. The physician who relies heavily on laboratory tests builds in a delay in treatment which is often critical.

Weather and climate do have a great influence on our sanogenetic forces and thus alters our health and wellbeing. Take spring, for example, when one has the maximum chance of falling ill. Fresh fruit and vegetables are fewer in number (the previous summer's stock has run out). As the ground thaws, the hibernating germs and viruses are released into the air, the moulds fly, pollens are released and, on top of all this, the body is trying to adapt from cold weather to a warmer climate. All this leads to susceptibility to various diseases but if the adaptogenic power in your body is good, you will not suffer from hay fever, flu etc.

BIORHYTHMS

In nature we see seasonal cycles in 12-month periods (spring returns every 12 months) and the world changes with this cycle. In the temperate climate every autumn the leaves change their colour and are shed. The day and night cycle changes our bodily hormones, as a result of which sleep and wakefulness are produced.

On New Year's Day in the Indian calendar, first of Baishak, people harvest wheat in the Punjab. The wheat is ripe on exactly the same day every year. After the Festival of Colours (Holi), the heatwave starts and the temperature rises steadily. After the Festival of Lights (Diwali), the temperature begins to drop as winter approaches. Why do these festivals coincide so strikingly with changes in nature? The Indian calendar is so astronomically accurate, marking the full moon, new moon, and so on, and it is amazing how it reflects the movements and changes of the sun and moon.

Biorhythms and the body

Similarly the mind has its ups and downs in a rhythmic fashion. Normally the physical cycle lasts for 23 days. This means that approximately every 23 days we are going to have a period of 'high' and a period of 'low' energy. Many of us notice the periods of high and low in our physical state but few realise that this pattern is cyclical. Likewise there are cycles of mental well-being lasting for 28 days and the emotional cycle lasts for 25 days on an average, though with individual variations. These cycles are strange but true. Soviet scientists worked on thousands of individuals before drawing them up. They are called biorhythms.

There are numerous examples of biorhythms in our body. The menstrual cycle is an obvious one. Bouts of loss of appetite, increased sexual urge, fatigue or sleep disturbances follow a rhythmic pattern. In a boarding school nearly all the girls have periods around the same time. Mothers and daughters do too. Biorhythms are 'contagious'. In families where the husband is stressed, the entire family is also under the weather. Most of us brush this aside as coincidental but when recorded over a period of time, their occurrences show a rhythmic pattern.

I was told that foreign visits of Soviet President Brezhnev were planned according to his biorhythms. He was generally a physically weak person in the later years of his life. A period of time that coincided with the 'high' of physical, psychological and emotional well-being was obviously the best time to carry out an important duty. Unfortunately all three factors rarely peak at the same time but they can peak near to each other. The opposite can also happen and one can have all three parameters on the low side at the same time. Should that happen one would be devastated with complete lack of mental and physical stamina. Again this is a rare phenomenon, basically because the cycles are of different duration and the probability of them all having their peaks or dips at the same time is low.

Many believe that these biorhythms are determined by the position of the moon and the planets. After all, the moon affects the high and low tides. It is therefore possible, in principle, that the biorhythms of the body can be affected by the moon and planets. Perhaps astrologers studied these laws over thousands of years to formulate their principles of prophecy. This raises the question, however, of why everybody doesn't react in the same way at the same time in accordance with the planetary positions. Perhaps our constitutional structure has the clue to this. We are all the same in structure, yet not the same when it comes to our constitution.

Biorhythm charts can be used to select moments when a person is likely to produce peak performance and avoid times when he is likely to have a very 'depressing' state of physical and mental well-being. This is possible because these cycles can be charted many years in advance.

Thus sportsmen will perform their best when they are in 'peak' form and do badly when they are not. It is no wonder that the top golf or tennis players sometimes play badly even though they are in 'top' physical form. Tiger Woods and Pete Sampras certainly do not win every competition. This is happening in all spheres of life and we are not aware of it.

Biorhythm chart

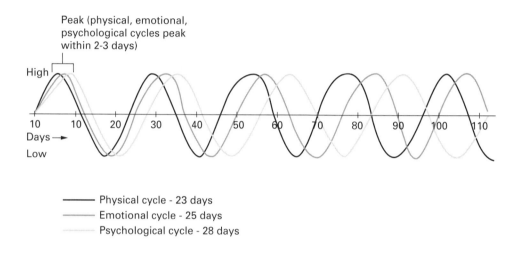

Peak (physical, emotional, psychological cycles peak within 2-3 days)

——— Physical cycle - 23 days
——— Emotional cycle - 25 days
········· Psychological cycle - 28 days

How biorhythms affect organs

Every function in our body has a cyclical pattern and its own rhythm. There is a short 24-hour rhythm and there is a longer monthly rhythm and a yearly rhythm. It is generally accepted that there are diurnal (solar), monthly (lunar) and yearly (planetary) cycles in nature. These changes in nature bring about changes in the body's organs and their functions, and these changes can be recorded and observed.

The ancient Chinese philosophers and medical practitioners explained biorhythms very well. According to ancient Chinese physicians, each organ or system had its own biorhythm. Here are some examples. The liver is most active between 1 a.m. and 3 a.m. but least active between 1 p.m. and 3 p.m., exactly 12 hours later. The gall bladder is in peak form between 11 p.m. and 1 a.m. and is least active between 11 a.m. and 1 p.m. The lungs are very active between 3 a.m. and 5 a.m. and the colon is active between 5 a.m. and 7 a.m. These biorhythmic peaks may look very arbitrary but in reality they have been established through centuries of observation and study.

Today we have some statistics which may just back up this hypothesis on biorhythms of organs. Most people get gall bladder colics between 11 p.m. and 1 a.m., the period during which this organ is very active. Most people who die in their sleep die because of thrombosis of the brain or heart arteries. The liver controls the clotting system of the body because it manufactures most of the enzymes. Could it be that it is the peak in activity in the liver between 1 a.m. and 3 a.m. that causes thrombosis of arteries to take place at that time? One needs to study this in detail – for the time being this is just an interesting hypothesis supported by powerful statistics. Most people who suffer from bronchitis or asthma have severe bouts of coughing or wheezing between 3 a.m. and 5 a.m., the period during which the lungs have peak performance. As soon as people wake up in the morning they have an urge to go to the toilet to clear their bowels, which presumably are in 'peak' form between 5 a.m. and 7 a.m. Similarly most people get 'heart attacks' between 7 a.m. and 9 a.m. as they get ready to go to work and, as it happens, the heart has its 'peak' in the biorhythmic cycle during this time. All these occurences sound very coincidental but ancient Chinese physicians observed them.

Chinese physicians use biorhythms in pulse diagnosis. Through pulse analysis they are able to tell the activity of various organs and their functioning. Thus a patient who has abnormally high activity in the gall bladder when the pulse is checked at 11 a.m., will be diagnosed as having inflammation in the gall bladder, because at 11 a.m. this organ is meant to have very low energy according to the biorhythmic chart.

Just like the various organs the psyche or the mind also has its biorhythms, which are daily, monthly and yearly cycles. Daily cycles can be explained by sleep and wakefulness. One is alert and active during the day, sleepy and sluggish at night. Monthly cycles are represented by the psychological and emotional biorhythms already discussed. Yearly cycles are represented by individuals feeling well during certain times of the year and miserable at others. Most people in the temperate zone feel best during the summer when there is plenty of sunshine, flowers, fresh fruits and vegetables, whereas in the sub-tropical zones people feel best during the winter months when the climate is moderate. Avicenna, the great Persian physician, explained these yearly psychic changes in his epic *Canon of Medicine*.

When the body is diseased or suffering mental illness these natural biorhythmic cycles get altered too. Mental patients in the psychiatric hospital sleep all day, waking up around 3 p.m. quite alert. Their day starts then. They become very active and chatty throughout the night. When I did duty in a psychiatric hospital, we used to have a tough time trying to bring law and order in the ward at night. All the patients, some of whom would even have taken sleeping tablets, wandered about talking to themselves or their mates and created pandemonium in the ward. It was only in the early hours of the morning that they would return to their beds one by one and drop off to sleep. Most mental illnesses start off with insomnia and lack of sleep. Potential patients lose sleep and feel very drowsy throughout the day, thus struggling to keep awake at work and showing signs of abnormal behaviour.

The yearly cycle in mental illness is clearly seen in the case of schizophrenia. In the temperate zone acute attacks take place in springtime while in warm countries they occur during the winter months. This is an abnormal pathological biorhythm and should not be confused with the normal biorhythms which have been described earlier.

Biorhythms and cycles in nature (seasons, climate) are one and the same phenomenon of the universal law. It clearly shows that everything is linked. It is therefore very important to look around us, at the climate and environment that surrounds us, to find clues for many of our ailments. Mental illnesses are the most direct example of this link. Lunatics were not named after the phases of the moon by accident.

In a physiology course the professors try to explain all these things as much as possible with the help of fundamental science, but they leave a topic when it goes beyond explanation. We have to understand that there are forces within us that are beyond explanation by science. We have to respect this and not treat the body with an entirely scientific attitude. If you can get away from this constraint you can begin to understand the physis as something much deeper than can be analysed mathematically, chemically or physically. Above all, we must accept that individuals are different and need different diagnosis and treatment.

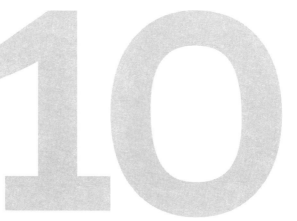

Chapter 10

CARRYING OUT AN MOT

So far in this book we have focused on how to be healthy – not just free of disease but as healthy as you can be. In order to achieve this you need to stop from time to time to analyse yourself. I call this My Own Testing, or MOT. You should do it regularly, because health is such an important aspect of our life, it determines our well-being, our thought processes, the level of our energy system, our work and family life. It is very important that you introduce certain checks, just as you do with your car. In practice we already do a routine servicing of ourselves by taking recreation: we play sports and go for holidays, which are meant to re-create our energy. This, however, is not an analysis.

Many of us go as far as having an annual medical check-up but, in the majority of cases, this fails to determine our state of health. It only shows whether infections are present and whether the body constants, the homeostasis, are right or not – blood pressure, blood count, cholesterol level, heart function and so on. Because our body has got this phenomenal capacity to keep these constants in balance within ourselves, very rarely do these parameters change. Some companies send their executives to very expensive clinics, spending up to $50,000, and the result boils down to very little. It confirms the client is free from disease but tells you little or nothing about his or her state of health. It does not tell you, for example, if he or she is fit to take the stress of company management. Insurance companies insist on medicals, too. They will have to pay out if you fall sick, though it is surprising that they too put so little emphasis on finding out how healthy you are.

The MOT I recommend consists of a series of questions:

1 What is your weight and has it changed? Has your waist size changed?
2 Has your sleep pattern changed? More important, are you tired during the day? This checks the level of energy.
3 Are you evacuating properly? Do you have excess flatulence or gas? Do you have excessive acid or heartburn?
4 Do the joints hurt? Does any part of your spine need attention?
5 Do you have dandruff? Does the skin around your nose and face look a bit scruffy or flaky?
6 Are there any swellings?
7 How do you smell? Do your urine or stools smell foul?

Once you ask these questions it will be clear to you whether your systems are functioning properly or not.

Then you should ask yourself some questions about your mental health:

- Have you been more irritable than usual?
- Have you been slightly depressed, a bit more anxious, are you getting panic attacks?
- Do you think you're doing enough to maintain calmness inside yourself?

Then ask yourself about your regimen or lifestyle:

- How many times per week are you eating out?
- Are you eating or drinking anything in excess?
- How much water are you drinking?
- Do you rely on supplements?
- Have you been doing exercises?

Then you can go a little further into self-diagnosis. Examine your tongue, read your pulse, perhaps read your blood pressure. I recommend elderly people should buy a blood pressure machine and do this.

These are the self-checks you need to carry out. It will give you enough information to answer the question 'How healthy are you?': very healthy, healthy, borderline-healthy, borderline-sick or sick. Let me stress, however, that the purpose of these checks is to determine your state of health, not whether you are sick. I will deal with that in the next section.

Body measurements

Weight

Excess weight puts stress on the lower back, the joints, the discs and the heart. It is also an indicator of plaque formation in the arteries and joints, lack of exercise, indulgence and ill-health. If you have excess weight the heart has to work that much harder to supply oxygen and you need more energy to carry yourself around. If you are not doing exercises the muscles are not fit enough and the strain on the discs of the spine increases. The anti-gravitational force provided by the spinal muscles is overwhelmed. You are at risk of disc compressions, and injuries to the hip and knee joints. It could be a continuous strain on your body.

You need to know three things about your weight:
- What is your optimum weight?
- What is your normal weight?
- How much has it changed recently?

It is very important to try to maintain your optimum weight.

There is a quick rule of thumb to calculate your optimum weight. Subtract 100 from your height in centimetres and that is roughly your ideal weight in kilograms. (If your height is 160 cm and you take away 100, it gives you an ideal weight of 60 kg; if your height is 180 cm your ideal weight would be 80 kg.)

The next step is to find out what your normal weight is. Just take an average over the past few weighings. If there is a significant difference between your normal weight and what it should be, you need to do something about it. But remember, there can be individual variations. A muscular person's ideal weight could be above the average, that of a woman with osteoporosis might be below average. Furthermore, if you take a lot of exercise much of any 'excess' weight could be the muscle and that is perfectly healthy.

If you are doing regular exercises, you may be able to cope with some excess weight (within reason) without back tension, breathlessness when you walk upstairs or lethargy (especially in the early morning when you feel sluggish). If all these physical signs are OK, your weight is OK. A 10 per cent increase on your ideal weight, however, is the danger limit. (So for a person whose ideal weight is 80 kg, 88 kg is the danger limit.) That's when the body will start to act up, especially the lower back – one of the commonest sites for weight-related problems.

Finally, if your recent weighings show an upward trend, then again you must take action. Sometimes, however, women over the age of 50 or 60, after losing weight (due to calcium loss in the bones), start putting it on again, only because they are gaining muscle and depositing calcium in the bones, especially if they exercise regularly. Weight loss is usually from water because usually we retain a lot of water. When I put people on healthy diets they lose weight quite rapidly in the first month or so. Then they plateau. The waist measurement may still reduce but not the weight. This is because the diet is combined with exercise, which creates muscles, and these weigh more than fat.

If you want to work out your ideal weight more scientifically, then follow the World Health Organisation (WHO) guidelines. According to WHO obesity is defined as a condition in which there is an excess of body fat. Body Mass Index (BMI), a calculation of build, is used to indicate the level of obesity. To work out your BMI, divide your weight (in kilograms) by the square of your height (in metres):

Metric weight (kg) $\div$ height (m^2) or:
Imperial weight (lb) x 704 $\div$ height ($inch^2$)
A normal BMI is in the range 18.5 – 24.9
You are overweight if your BMI is in the range 25.0 – 29.9
You are obese if your BMI is more than 30

WHO advises that generally, as a person's BMI increases, the risk of disease and other obesity-related conditions rises too. These include adult-onset diabetes, high blood pressure and high blood fats. (Interestingly, in Asia, the onset of these conditions occurs on average at a lower BMI, to such an extent that Regional Obesity Guidelines have had to be issued – another example of individuality ignored by the statisticians till recently.)

The death rate from heart disease shows that life expectancy shortens as the BMI rises above 23. It is said that up to half the population is at risk through obesity-related disorders. It has also been suggested that having 25 as the cut-off point for the 'normal' range of is politically motivated and if risks are evident over 23 then the cut-off point should be 23.

Whichever method you use, you should now be able to compare your ideal weight with what it actually is and take action to correct it if necessary. Read pages 46–74 for my advice on diet and exercise.

Other body measurements

There are four other body measurements you can do yourself. One is the **pulse rate**. Rest for a minute or two, then put three fingers (not your thumb) on your wrist just below the thumb on the outer side. Use a watch to check the number of beats per minute. It should be between 60 and 75. Lower is no problem, but higher than 80 is cause for concern. The pulse should be firm and steady, with no irregularities. Any sign of palpitations should be carefully watched.

Next measure your **waist**, though your clothing should tell you if it has grown. Again, we are looking for changes here, and a significant expansion should be checked.

Now put your hand on top of your abdomen and check your **breathing rate**. It should be about 16 breaths per minute. If you are hyperventilating it will be more. Relax, try not to be conscious of the breathing, let it be natural. It is not a problem if it is slower than 16. Pages 57–58 give advice on controlling your breathing and there are breathing exercises on pages 64–65.

Finally, if you have a **blood pressure** meter (they are not expensive and quite accurate), check the reading from time to time. When you are relaxed it should be between 120/70 and 135/85 if you are under 40 years old. In this case both high (over 140) and low (below 65) are cause for concern. Blood pressure tends to rise with age. This is normal. At age 70, 150/90 is OK. If you have high blood pressure, turn to pages 142–149 for advice on treatment.

Energy

How much do you **sleep**? Years ago we used to need eight hours sleep, now because of the increase in stress levels, it has generally gone down to six. What is important is the quality of your sleep. That may depend on your lifestyle. Do you work late, or get involved in problems in the evening? A continuous sleep is not essential and it can be averaged. If you get three really good nights' sleep in a week it doesn't really matter if the other nights are restless or wakeful to some extent. But if interrupted sleep causes tiredness or lethargy in the day then you have some catching-up to do – there is a problem. As long as you get a reasonable total, to which an afternoon siesta may be added, then there should be no problem. Insomnia is a problem only when it affects daytime performance. Some people get away with less sleep.

Watch the pattern – has it changed recently? This may be a result of stress. Three hours per night instead of the usual six or seven indicates something is wrong. Look for dark circles round the eyes. They will tell you whether you have been sleeping well or superficially.

Fatigue is one of the most injurious conditions to health. Without energy you are done for. It is like a power failure in the body. The liver will not function well, your absorption, circulation and kidney function will be poor, your muscles will not be toned, you will be prone to depression. Ask yourself how bright you are when you wake up. Do you leap out of bed with vitality or ease out like a snail from its shell? What about an hour after lunch? Are you still full of beans? How exhausted are you at night? Do you feel the day's activities have really taken their toll, or are you still game for more? It is OK to be aware that your energy is limited and you have to care for it, to accept some tiredness at night, but regular exhaustion is bad.

Digestive system

It is not necessary to **evacuate** in the mornings. Any time of day is OK. But within 24 hours you should move the bowels. Mild constipation slows you down even if it does not cause a complete blockage. You should not have to force it. Give yourself plenty of time. Don't hurry. Drink a couple of glasses of water in the morning to stimulate the bowels.

Check your urine. It should be clear or pale yellow with no strong smell. If it is very yellow you are not drinking enough water. If it is strong smelling you may have taken an excess of vitamins (particularly B) or protein. Do you have a burning sensation as you pass urine? Are you getting up too often in the night? Similar telltale signs are foul-smelling stools. If you have any of these symptoms you may need to see your doctor, but try Regimen Therapy first.

Do you experience excessive **flatulence,** burping or passing a lot of wind? By excessive I mean enough for you to notice it as too often. Do you have bloating in the abdomen, are the belt and waistline of clothes getting tighter? This could be caused by stress, eating too fast, producing too much acid, irregular meals, taking a lot of the wrong foods or drink (e.g. spicy food, nuts, white wine, champagne, fizzy drinks). Try reducing your acid-producing foods and do some relaxation every day. Incidentally, when you move from rest, the abdominal muscles press on the stomach walls and push gas up. Some resultant burping is all right, but not in excess and it should not contain an acid taste. Chapter 5 (pages 46–54) gives more advice on diet. Relaxation techniques are described on pages 74–75. Treatment for gastritis (excess acidity) is explained on pages 207–209.

Analyse your **breath**. Blow from deep down into your palm and sniff. If you get a rotten egg or ammonia type of smell there is putrefaction going on in your gums or your stomach. Gum boils, gingivitis or pyorrhoea can cause bad smells through the secretion of pus. Oral hygiene is important. The vapours from the stomach also come up continuously into the mouth. A bad smell could be caused by eating protein in excess or failing to digest properly. If there is a sweet or acetone (nail varnish) smell you are eating too many carbohydrates. The smell is caused by excess yeast and fermenting alcohol in the stomach. These are the two main smells, though a physician can detect a lot more.

Analyse your **drinking** habits. How much water are you drinking? It is important to flush the system. You need six to eight glasses a day. No chemical reaction can take place in the body without water. So if you are dehydrated the cells become shrivelled and they do not function to their full capacity. Moreover, the build-up of toxins in the tissue retards chemical processes and there will be a further build-up of toxins.

Alcohol puts stress on the liver. Alcohol also dehydrates you in the long run. The body tries to expel the alcohol by increasing the heart and breathing rate so, even if you have been drinking water as well, ultimately you are not left with anything like the intake you thought you had. (It's like taking a hot bath – it stops the natural heating of the body, so when you get out you are cold. Same with alcohol. You take a drink and it has to be eliminated. The rate of elimination is so fast it dehydrates you.) Spirits are worse since they have so little water of their own it has to come from somewhere else.

The main difficulty with alcohol is its addictive property. Irregular drinking is OK. A few glasses at the weekend or at the odd party are OK. Three glasses of wine a week do no harm at all, while three glasses a day are almost certain to produce digestive, arthritic and addictive problems. Wine has a lot of fungus in it (spirits don't), so it produces gas and sensitises you to fungi. Cheap wine in general is worse than good-quality wine. On the whole, however, there is no way people can completely control themselves when taking a substance with an addictive property. So three glasses a week usually leads to three glasses a day. As a physician I have to warn people that regular intake of alcohol, particularly cheap hooch, is dangerous. They may still do it. It's the same with smoking. Every packet spells out that it is injurious to health. Who takes notice of it? Amazingly few people.

You can check for digestive problems by examining the state of your tongue. Stick out your tongue in front of a mirror and look for the following signs:

1 Tongue with impressions of teeth. Signs of gastritis with acidity.
2 Tongue of a person consuming excess carbohydrates (sweets, chocolate etc).
3 Tongue of a person with constipation or sluggish bowel movements.
4 Tongue with uniform greyish coating and slight reddish irritation on the sides. Signifies chronic acidity problem (high stomach acid).
5 Tongue showing purple or dark patches indicating chronic anaemia (past or current).
6 Tongue showing evidence of 'gut fermentation' or mild yeast overgrowth in the abdomen. Patient may complain of flatulence, cramps etc.
7 Also known as 'geographical tongue'. Indicates signs of liver malfunction or sluggish liver. Could also indicate psoriasis.
8 Ulcerations on the tongue. Shows signs of severe fungal or yeast overgrowth in the abdomen. Deficiency of vitamin B[1]
9 Severe gastritis or stomach ulcer.
10 Dehydrated tongue (slightly shrivelled) with a shiny coating of saliva. Sign of low water consumption.

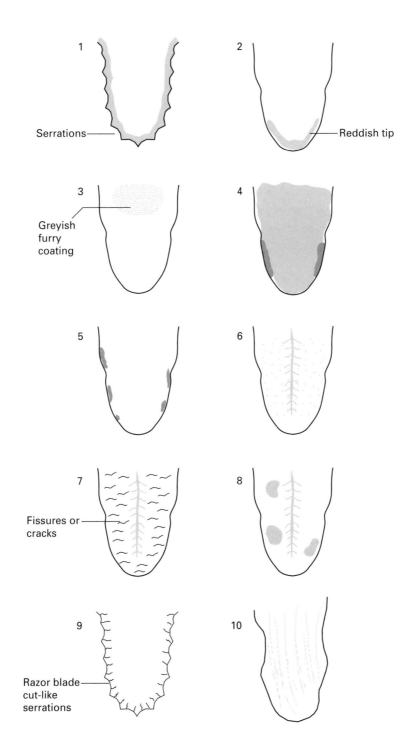

1 Serrations

2 Reddish tip

3 Greyish furry coating

4

5

6

7 Fissures or cracks

8

9 Razor blade cut-like serrations

10

Musculo-skeletal system

Do you have any aches and pains in the **back**? If not, ask someone to press along the spine, along the neck, upper back and lower back. Press a couple of centimetres either side of the back bone. Test for any area of tenderness. Stress tightens the muscles up and brings the discs closer together, so the spine shrinks. If you have not done the correct sort of exercises, if you have had too much strain, had too many air flights, with changes of bed, dehydration on the plane (which also tightens muscles), then your spine is in trouble. Treatment for spinal problems is described on pages 158–169.

Then feel your **joints**. Look for aches and pains, tender areas. If you drive a lot, write or use keyboards much of the time, then feel the area between the elbow and the wrist. Squeeze the **muscles** and let go several times on both sides. If you find sore spots, massage them. Try to eliminate them. They can ultimately lead to pain in the elbow and repetitive strain injury. Do the shoulders too. Check the state of your calves. If they are in spasm there is a chance you might get clots. The spasms cause resistance to blood flow. Massage them, squeeze and let go, or you can press with a circular motion on specific sore spots. These sore spots mean the muscle has been overused or injured or has an accumulation of lactic acid. If you massage or stretch, they will usually go away. If they don't go away you need to see a physician. It could be referred pain from discs of the spine. Pages 76–82 give you more information about how to look after your muscles and how to massage.

Another test you can do is to lie flat on your back on the floor. The moment you lie down the curvature of the spine is changed and there is a natural traction. If there are any trapped nerves or tissue you will feel it. You can also try bending forward and from side to side and twisting the neck as far as it will go each side. These movements also reveal spinal problems.

You can also search for sore spots by pressing quite hard all over your hands and the soles of your feet. If you feel any soreness, check with the reflexology charts I have included here and you may find an indication of some organ not functioning properly. Don't scoff at this. The procedures are as old as medicine itself and have been proven to work from time immemorial.

Reflexology charts

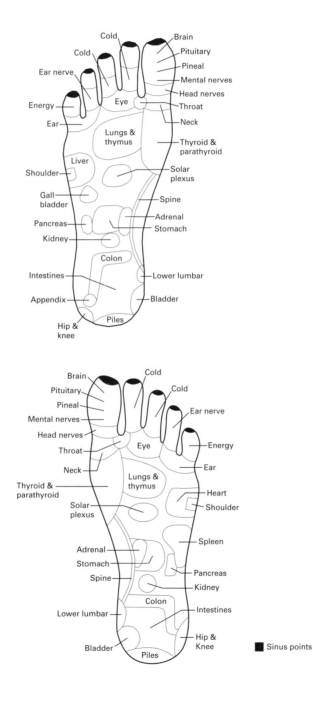

Outer surface of the body

There are two types of toxin, water soluble and fat soluble (most organic substances are either water- or fat soluble). Water soluble toxins come out in sweat. The skin will be oily if there are fat-soluble toxins. It can also become scaly and rough. Dandruff is an example. If you have yeast in your system or you have been drinking too much, the skin round the nose will change its colour because of the toxins that are being continually secreted. So the **face** is a good place to see evidence of toxins. Men should look for 'barber's itch'. When you shave you can get small dots around the chin. This is actually seborrheic dermatitis. The sebaceous glands are throwing out too many fat-soluble toxins. If water-soluble toxins are being secreted then you can have irritation and itchiness of the skin, with red, eczema-like patches.

If you notice problems like this, cut out yeast and sugar products from your diet and reduce your intake of fat, citrus fruits, coffee and alcohol. On one day each week drink only water and eat only vegetable soup and fruit. Soak $1/_4$ teaspoon of Kadu powder (Black Helibore) in a cup of water at night and drink it next morning on an empty stomach. Homoeopathic remedies are also very useful for treating these types of toxic rash.

Then look at the **nails**. Spots generally indicate some deficiency such as calcium or zinc. A line across all the nails indicates you have had a fever or chronic inflammation of some kind during the last four months (the time it takes a nail to grow from bottom to top). The position of the line enables you to calculate when the condition occurred (see diagram b). If such lines appear repeatedly there is something wrong. Indentations and whitish roughness are signs of fungal infection and you should look to your diet. Pages 230–233 give advice on diet and treatment for fungal infections of the skin. Check your nails against the diagrams opposite.

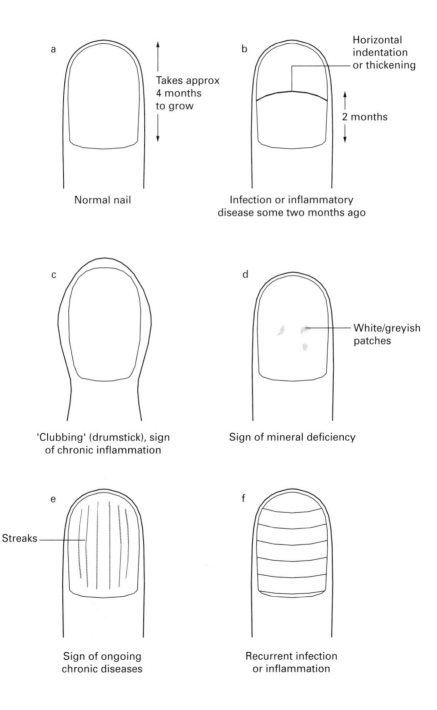

a

Takes approx
4 months
to grow

Normal nail

b

Horizontal
indentation
or thickening

2 months

Infection or inflammatory
disease some two months ago

c

'Clubbing' (drumstick), sign
of chronic inflammation

d

White/greyish
patches

Sign of mineral deficiency

e

Streaks

Sign of ongoing
chronic diseases

f

Recurrent infection
or inflammation

Check if you are losing hair. If **hair loss** has suddenly increased then either there is some deficiency of minerals or vitamins, or a restriction of the blood flow to the scalp.

Now you should look at your **eyes** in a mirror. A trained physician can tell a great deal from the appearance of the iris of the eye, so much so that there is a whole science devoted to it, called iridology (see charts opposite). I am not expecting this of you. You can, however, look at the colour of the sclera (the whites). If you are tense the small blood vessels will be slightly shrivelled. If you have a lot of toxins in the system or you have been stressed for a long period of time, then the shrivelled capillaries will have burst. If this has happened recently you will see a reddish colour in the sclera, which will look slightly bloodshot (see diagram a). That means that fresh blood has seeped out of the blood vessels. Over a period of time the iron in the blood is converted into ferrous chloride or ferrous oxide, which is brownish red in colour. You could say your eyes have gone rusty (see diagram b). If this has happened you are not 100 per cent healthy. You must take action. Pages 182–190 give advice on managing and treating stress.

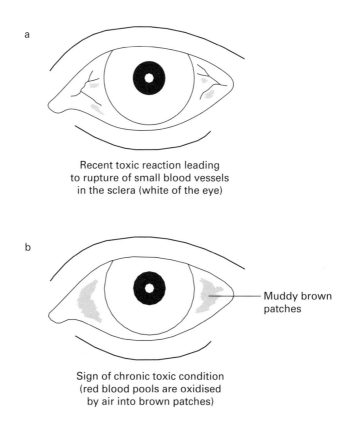

a

Recent toxic reaction leading
to rupture of small blood vessels
in the sclera (white of the eye)

b

Muddy brown
patches

Sign of chronic toxic condition
(red blood pools are oxidised
by air into brown patches)

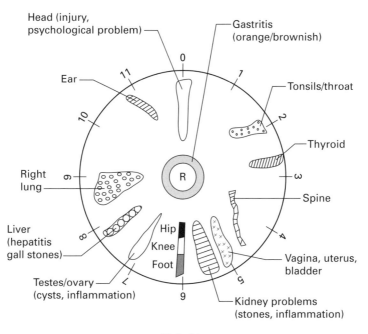

Right iris

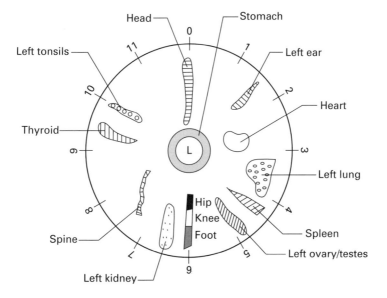

Left iris

Changes in the marked zones indicate disease or inflammation (chronic or acute) of the referred organs or systems.

Look for **swellings** in and around the feet. The skin has a soft part and a hard part. Press on the soft areas. If there is a swelling, when you press, indentations remain momentarily. It is called pitting. Then you know you are retaining water, or the kidneys are below par, or the heart is not pumping very well, depending on your age. If you are over 70 the likely cause is the heart. Look for puffiness around the eyes, particularly in the early morning. Rings on the fingers may feel a bit tight. See pages 237–245 for advice on treatment of heart problems.

Finally how does your **body smell**? A strong odour usually means you have been eating too much protein. Personal hygiene is important. Take enough baths and showers. Look after your oral/dental hygiene. Hygiene after sexual contact is important. If you have long hair, wash it frequently. Long hair can cause your eyes to itch. Long nails take more looking after too.

Mental health

Ask yourself, have I been unusually irritable recently? Have I had mild depression, or suffered anxiety or panic attacks with hyperventilation or heavy breathing? Have I been able to maintain calmness in the face of stress? Have I been yawning a lot? What about short-term memory? Have I been forgetting what happened an hour before? The answers to these questions should reveal your state of mental health and whether you need a holiday. Pages 182–190 also offer advice on dealing with stress.

Lifestyle

Have I maintained a sensible regimen? How often have I eaten out? Were the meals late? Did I drink a lot or too much? In general, have I been overindulging? What have I been eating in excess – coffee, chocolates, wine, beer or bread? Have I had enough vegetables to meet my daily requirements for vitamins and minerals? Have I drunk enough water each day (six to eight glasses). Have I been taking supplements? Have I kept on one variety for a long time? Should I be changing to something else, or having a break altogether and relying on my diet? Have I had enough exercise, both daily with breathing exercises (such as yoga) and sports? If you are a hyperactive type, do exercises that calm you down and vice versa. It is quite easy to lead a healthy life without a strict regimen, though if your health is suffering the strict regimen may well be the answer.

I have summarised the questions in this chapter in the form of the short questionnaire which follows. Answer this, to yourself only, as honestly as you can. It will give you a good pointer to your state of health. Remember tolerance levels. The purpose of the questionnaire is not to highlight any weakness, but to assess the state of your physis as a totality. Only the total is meaningful.

If the result shows room for improvement, if it shows something is wrong, then the Lifestyle Programme would be the ideal cure. Although ideally you should do it throughout life, I know this is usually impracticable. As a guide, however, after a festive season such as Christmas you should force yourself for a month or six weeks to do a Lent-like adherence to the Lifestyle Programme. Use your holidays, not to live it up but to balance things up. People so often do the opposite. They live a life of excess in eating and drinking and then do it even more on holidays and put on weight. They often come back sick. Some do a bit of exercise – swimming, surfing, walking, golf – but the sensible thing is to do the diet as well. It is very important to use your holidays for recreation – re-creating energy. You need the break. Too many people come back needing another holiday to counteract the effect of the first. My patients that come trekking in the Himalayas find it strenuous and ascetic. The results are outstanding. Patients want to come back again and again.

Apart from holidays, go on a liquid – (non-alcoholic) – diet once or twice a month, or even fast for a day. This is very beneficial. Take massages from time to time, especially if you have been travelling or not doing exercises or sports.

If you do all this you are keeping your physis on guard – all the time. You are not taking it for granted, saying 'I'll look after it when it fails', or, worst of all, saying 'It's not my responsibility. I leave all that sort of thing to the doctor!'

My Own Testing
Tick the appropriate box

Measurements	Just right	So so	Not normal
1 Weight	☐	☐	☐
2 Pulse (shouldn't be over 80)	☐	☐	☐
3 Waist	☐	☐	☐

Physical factors	Seldom	Sometimes	Frequently
1 Sleep badly?	☐	☐	☐
2 Tired: On waking up?	☐	☐	☐
1 hour after lunch?	☐	☐	☐
End of day?	☐	☐	☐
3 Have trouble evacuating properly?	☐	☐	☐
4 Urine smelly or yellow?	☐	☐	☐
5 Foul-smelling stools?	☐	☐	☐
6 Excess flatulence or burping?	☐	☐	☐
7 Much acidity?	☐	☐	☐
8 Foul-smelling breath?	☐	☐	☐
9 Tongue: Thick coating, redness, cracks, ulcers?	☐	☐	☐
10 Joints hurt, particularly spine?	☐	☐	☐
11 Scruffy or flaky skin?	☐	☐	☐
12 Itchiness?	☐	☐	☐
13 Swellings?	☐	☐	☐
14 Dandruff?	☐	☐	☐

Mental	Seldom	Sometimes	Frequently
1 Irritable periodically?	☐	☐	☐
2 Depression, anxiety, panic attacks?	☐	☐	☐
3 Maintain calmness?	☐	☐	☐
4 Yawn a lot?	☐	☐	☐
5 Poor short-term memory?	☐	☐	☐

Regimen

		A	B	C
1	How often eat out?	☐	☐	☐
2	Overeat?	☐	☐	☐
3	Too much chocolate, wine, bread, coffee?	☐	☐	☐
4	Too few vegetables?	☐	☐	☐
5	Not enough exercise?	☐	☐	☐
6	Drink too little water?	☐	☐	☐
7	Rely on supplements?	☐	☐	☐

Totals

        A   **B**   **C**

How did you do?

Calculate $2 \times A + B$ = ...
40 or more: you are healthy
50 or more: you are very healthy – congratulations
60: you cheated

If your score is less than 40 you should seriously consider changes in your lifestyle. If it is less than 30 you need to visit an integrated medical physician, probably a naturopath or complementary medical practitioner, if the former is not available.

Part III
WHEN THINGS
GO WRONG

Chapter 11

RESTORING HEALTH

So far I have been describing the most important part of medicine, the maintenance and optimising of health. If this were 100 per cent successful there would be no need for treatment of disease or hospitals and national healthcare budgets could be decimated. This is not a perfect world, however, and things do go wrong. So in the second half of the book I am going to join the National Disease Service (which is a more accurate name for the NHS) and focus on restoring health.

Just as health results from the careful balancing of the body's systems (described in Chapter 3), so diseases are the result of the lowering of the sanogenetic defences (physis), allowing pathogens to attack one or more of those systems, throwing them out of balance. How do we restore the balance and effect a cure? Do we boost the defences, or do we attack the pathogens? Do we treat the diseased, or the disease?

Immediately we have come to the parting of the ways. Conventional medicine, also known as allopathic medicine, treats the disease, often ignoring the individuality of the patient (the diseased) and even the cause in the blind rush to recreate normality. Integrated medicine treats the patient as an individual and a co-operative partner in the fight against the disease and the restoration of health.

The methods too are different. The word 'allopathic' comes from *allo* 'other' and *pathos* meaning 'disease'. In other words, conventional medicine introduces other pathogens, usually toxins (in the case of drugs like digoxin or chemotherapy, potentially lethal toxins) to counter the first (the disease). Integrated medicine adjusts the lifestyle of the patient (the diseased) to restore the defensive network and the balance of the systems to their healthy state. Conventional medicine therefore requires least effort from the patient who simply remains passive and takes the treatment, often allowing the body's own efforts, such as the secretion of natural steroids, to be suppressed. Integrated medicine is hard on the patient because it demands his or her full co-operation and effort to build up the physis, often by sheer hard work, but with a far higher ultimate reward – health.

To illustrate my point I am including in the following chapters guidance on conditions relating to each of the systems discussed in Parts 1 and 2, with one or more examples in each case of a disease centred primarily in that system. I will explain the symptoms and treatment recommended by integrated medicine and also explain where conventional medicine is appropriate and where it fails. Use this as a guideline only and be warned that these instructions are no way an open licence to self-treatment. Consult your doctor when you feel that safe methods like the Regimen Therapy are producing no results.

DIAGNOSIS

The first step in countering a disease is diagnosis. My method of diagnosis and treatment is similar to that of a traditional practitioner. When I saw these traditional physicians at work, I was convinced that their *modus operandi* was the best way forward. They had very powerful methods of diagnosis. I was taught the traditional Chinese method of pulse diagnosis, in which the physician places three fingers on the radial artery in the wrist and senses the form of the beats. Originally the training for this started by asking a student to feel a human hair beneath a fine silk cloth, then between two cloths, then three and so on, up to seven. When the apprentice could sense the hair through seven such cloths he was regarded as fit to train. Later, thin paper was used. This may seem to be expecting a lot, but when you consider what a blind person can detect when reading braille it is not so unusual. In the chinese school students are taught to sense up to 28 variations in the pulse, indicating problems in various organs, though I only mastered 17.

In addition to this a physician should carefully examine a patient from the moment they enter the door, observing how they look, sit, stand, talk. It is worth looking the patient in the eye or standing close to them for a few moments to establish communication and empathy.

Because of the mass of tiny blood vessels behind the eye, the iris also reveals a wealth of information about the body's state of health, so much so that there is a subject devoted to it, called iridology. The Russians pioneered the development of this science from traditional practice and that is where I learned the art. As I mentioned in Chapter 10 you can also learn a lot, especially about the digestive system, by examining the tongue. Finally, using a special instrument you can detect the state of many of the organs in the body by testing the acupuncture points on the ears. The instruments measure surface conductivity and are hyperactive on points representing diseased (or irritated) organs.

Application of these skills earned me in time a reputation as a very accurate diagnostician and this fact is now well known amongst my patients and colleagues. I was once challenged to diagnose six patients brought into the lecture hall of the Kenyan Medical Research Institute (KEMRI) in Nairobi, with the auditorium filled with doctors. Without the patients or me speaking a word I diagnosed them all correctly, causing quite a stir among the staff. If you can tell your patients what is wrong with them before they have uttered a word, it helps enormously in establishing their confidence in you.

I firmly believe that you should not treat without a definite diagnosis in mind. If making such a diagnosis is difficult on a patient's first visit, I take my time and ponder over it until the next time I see them. In the meantime I recommend the **Regimen Therapy**, which does no harm anyway. If a detective has a suspect, he doesn't always dive in and arrest him, he finds out more about him. He watches and observes. A physician should be like a detective, looking for clues, analysing them and then making deductions, taking ample time to find out the exact causes of the various complaints and symptoms. All too often a patient's records show that the diagnosis has changed regularly, suggesting premature diagnosis in the first place and probably unnecessary tests and medication.

When a patient comes with a large number of complaints and has many symptoms, in the case of a chronic ailment, you have to carefully compartmentalise them into different sections – physical, psychological, emotional and so on – and then try to look for links between them and the telltale signs. Very often no links are found and that is when you have to wait and see. If the patient is a hypochondriac, their complaints will not match the symptoms or the findings of the physician. That is quite easy to establish and you have to deal with that situation. However, the majority of such cases are genuine and you have to apply your knowledge and experience to draw a final conclusion on the diagnosis. The advantage of recommending the Regimen Therapy during the observation period in a chronic case is that many of the symptoms and complaints disappear and you are left with fewer symptoms to work with. It's like moving into an empty house. The first thing you have to do is to clear away the cobwebs and the dirt so you can see what it really looks like.

A very talented artist came to see me once with complaints of fatigue, flatulence, occasional diarrhoea, lack of periods, dry skin, aches and pains in the body, insomnia, frequent thirst and occasional headaches. She seemed very focused, slightly irritable, and looked slim and healthy. I examined her pulse and looked at her tongue. Except for some irritation in the colon and slight low blood pressure there were no objective findings. Even her hormonal levels were within normal range. Yet this woman suffered so much. I first put her on Regimen Therapy to try to find out more about the cause of the symptoms. Within a month her fatigue improved and she had less flatulence but the other symptoms remained unchanged. I could not find any telltale signs that would give me the clue to her ailment. She complained that the treatment was not helping her much and this put me under great pressure to find a cause for the various symptoms. I began to focus on the colon, as the tongue and pulse diagnosis indicated that there was something wrong. One day I asked her to write down the things she ate. It became crystal clear that she did not eat any carbohydrates like bread, potato, pasta, rice or sugar but lived on proteins (egg, chicken, meat), fruits and vegetables only. On further inquiry it emerged that she took up to 30 laxative tablets a day to treat her constipation – a fact she had deliberately hidden from me. Then I began to investigate the matter further and the truth came out. She had been bulimic in the past and was always worried about her weight. She was obsessed that carbohydrates had high calories and helped to put on weight but the high-protein diet made her constipated, which often caused weight gain. She took the laxatives to combat that. Everything fell into place – she had a psychological problem that was hidden under the physical symptoms. It took me six weeks to solve the puzzle and make a diagnosis. Once I was sure what she had, I confronted her with the questions. This brought on denial from her side, as she insisted that the concern for her weight in an obsessive way was the main problem. She was frightened of any psychiatric help and she refused to face her own problem. This confirmed my diagnosis – obsessive-compulsive behaviour.

Most illnesses are multifactorial, meaning that several causative factors are involved with no apparent links between them. Common flu, for example, involves weakening of the physis, the presence of a virulent agent, the weakening of the lining of the nasal tract etc. resulting in headache, muscle ache, fatigue, all apparently unconnected. Conventional medicine has no convenient answer to a multifactorial illness: since drugs are designed to hit a particular pathogen, many symptoms require many drugs to hit each one. When a multifactorial disease is complex, like cancer or allergies, conventional medicine often has no answer at all. Integrated medicine, on the other hand, in boosting the body's own sanogenetic power, employs a healing agent which tackles all the factors. Hence general treatment in the form of Regimen Therapy, perhaps supplemented with a tonic, is in many cases the only answer, and it is one that individuals can apply the moment they feel ill, with absolutely no risk and a good chance of success.

Often, however, it is the single symptoms that cause concern, so the question arises, what diagnosis can you do yourself? Whole books have been written about this. Suffice it to say that symptoms of illness take on an importance when they cause discomfort, worry or concern. **Pain** is perhaps the most obvious. Some pains we can live with. Everybody has them from time to time. Pain (or stiffness) from exercise you ignore, as you do pain in the jaw through eating nuts. If you eat just before you pass your stools you may get a little cramp in your bowels, but you ignore it. If, however, pain is continuous or regular or it wakes you up at night you worry and you need to seek advice.

Another common symptom is **fever**. With fever you know you have to slow down. You don't go to work or school. Your heart rate and anxiety level go up, you are sluggish, your muscles and whole body ache. The symptoms restrict you. If you try to work through it you get dizzy and tired and you are sent home anyway. If it is a viral fever you have a runny nose, headache, muscular fatigue, cold congestion, slight irritation in the throat. This should be taken seriously. Regular fever at a particular time is cause for concern. If the fever is very high and the patient is delirious he needs a physician. In children and the elderly a fever lasting longer than 24 hours requires medical help and for other adults three to four days is the limit. Within these limits rest, warmth and a mild diet are sufficient. Don't try to reduce the temperature with drugs, unless it is very high (when the doctor should be involved anyway). The rise in temperature is the sanogenetic forces' way of limiting the pathogens which cannot survive at the higher temperature or simply cannot multiply. When the fever goes down it shows the sanogenetic forces have overcome but not completed their task.

Similarly with an abscess. The fact that it has burst (lysis) does not mean that healing is complete. The body has thrown out the toxins (pus) but still needs time to regenerate, to heal, so that there isn't a recurrence and you are not left with incomplete healing. After any infection recuperation is very important. The damage done to the physis has to be repaired.

DIFFERENT FORMS OF TREATMENT

I have made references to seeking medical help. As a simple rule of thumb: if the condition is acute (severe), go to a conventional doctor; if it is chronic (persistent) and conventional medicine failed at the onset, go to an integrated or complementary physician. In an integrated clinic you will first meet a gatekeeper, a skilled diagnostician and generalist who will direct you to the most appropriate treatment. In areas without such a clinic, however, the patient has to decide which form of treatment to seek or a well-informed GP can guide them. The gatekeeper in integrated medicine will give you the initial treatment plan of Regimen Therapy before sending you off to an appropriate specialist to complete the cure. Hithertho in complementary or alternative medical clinics the patient decides for himself or herself whether he wants acupuncture, homoeopathy etc. Nobody guides them. Here are some tips on which physician to go to when you are ill, having followed the basic principles of the Regimen Therapy.

Acupuncture

Acupuncture involves painless insertion of fine needles into trigger points in the skin, which stimulate the physis to focus on selected organs. Amongst other things it releases endorphins which are the body's own form of morphine and are excellent painkillers. It is used in hospitals to treat severe pain as in terminal cancer patients, and I use it for back pain, arthritic pains and migraine. Apart from its pain-killing properties it is used for stimulating energy, can help regulate the systems of the body (particularly the involuntary nervous system), and reduce inflammation, mild hypertension, panic attacks, insomnia, anxiety, itchiness, tinnitus, deafness, loss of smell, tingling and numbness in the fingers due to some neurological problem and loss of sensation. It can also be used to treat chronic fatigue as well as nerve-related conditions such as Bell's palsy, paralysis, stroke, stomach ulcers and double vision, to mention just a few examples.

Conventional medicine

At the Integrated Medical Centre we use conventional medicine as and when required. I would estimate that 30–35 per cent of our therapy is conventional: antibiotics, diuretics, painkillers, anti-histamine, occasionally tranquillisers, vitamins and minerals in infusions. We use the latter particularly for cancer therapies (because of poor appetite and the need to nourish the body with essentials), chronic fatigue syndrome (because of poor absorption) and during convalescence. In psychiatry we use psychological medicine, neurolinguistic programming (NLP), hypnosis, different types of psychological treatment and conventional medicines, depending on the acuteness of the disease.

Healing

Healing is a form of treatment that all doctors who touch their patients practise to some degree. There is a significant link between the physician and the physis of the patient when contact is made. When I have completed a period of, say, neck massage I feel strangely drained of energy. Though I recover quite quickly it is a very noticeable effect. There is no question in my experience that healing through the hands aids the physis. At the Integrated Medical Centre we use it very often in relief of chronic or unexplained panic attacks, pains, stress, chronic fatigue, multiple sclerosis (to some degree) and also for stroke. I would say that it brings about necessary change in the tissues to kick-start the healing process. The battery is flat, you give the car a push, jump-start it and off you go, charging up the battery.

Herbal remedies

Herbal remedies, (Ayurvedic, Chinese and Unani), are outstanding in the treatment of liver disorders, including hepatitis and particularly hepatitis C, for which conventional medicine is sadly weak. They can be used for chronic sinus problems, eczema (again, there is no conventional equivalent) and irritable bowel syndrome. The only remedy available for constipation, which is actually used by conventional medicine in its herbal form, is psyllium husk, or senna. We also use herbs for impotence, infertility, hypertension, toning up the heart and circulatory system, and tonics. There is not much money in herbal tonics so nowadays conventional medicine has turned to vitamin B complexes, which bring a much better return to the drug companies, but the herbal tonics are just as effective. Herbal remedies also work well for urinary infections and kidney stones, though not gall stones. Ayurvedic oils with anti-inflammatory properties are used for oil baths to help arthritis, chronic sciatica and chronic backache. Oil massage of the head has a soothing effect on the brain, a powerful psychotherapeutic effect and induces sleep.

Homoeopathy

Homoeopathy is an incredible science. A good homoeopathic physician holds a bunch of keys and knows exactly which key to fit into the lock of an ailment to open it. Homoeopathy is at its best with allergies, such as asthma, eczema and hayfever. It is also useful for problems of the mind, depression, anxiety, insomnia, warts, corns, benign growths, tonsillitis, acute flu (it works on the energy system of the body and builds up immunity), excess acidity, irritable bowel syndrome (if it is not connected with any food intolerances), rheumatoid arthritis and some auto-immune problems. In general it is most effective where the constitution or whole body needs to be built up.

Naturopathy

You can best treat many chronic ailments, such as eczema, asthma, gastritis, psoriasis, arthritis or liver disorders by naturopathy, that is fasting, diet, massage, water hydrotherapy and some juices, without the need for herbal, homoeopathic or any chemical medicines. Naturopathy relies solely on the physis to cure disease.

Nutritional medicine

Nowadays the soils are so depleted that they do not contain the microelements necessary for function of enzymes and for carrying out numerous chemical reactions. Vitamins and minerals are therefore used to ensure that the body is in a reasonable state, boosting the body's functions.

Osteopathy and Chiropractic

Osteopathy and chiropractic are used for any minor dislocation of joints. Although exercise and massage can normally clear such problems, patients usually want speedy relief. Maybe they can't walk, move or function in some way. Manipulation is often miraculous in its speed. Cranial osteopathy is a slow method of treatment but it improves circulation of blood and cerebral fluid to the brain, and so is well worth using on the principle that if the brain functions better the rest of the body functions better. People often ask the difference between osteopathy and chiropractic. To put it very simply, osteopathy focuses on muscles and bones and chiropractic only on bones. They both have their place in therapy.

Yoga

Specific therapeutic yoga is used for clearing sinuses and bowels, sports' injuries, backache, arthritis, insomnia, hypertension, bronchial asthma, panic attacks, infertility, stress, myopia, chronic fatigue etc. These exercises are recommended after doing the basic programme mentioned in Regimen Therapy.

The role of Regimen Therapy

Following the **Regimen Therapy** is an excellent way to build a foundation for treatment. The programme creates optimum nutrition (by regulation of digestion), improves circulation (through massage), removes physical and mental stress (through yoga), and generates well-being (through all three). Once the patient 'feels good' all the self-regulatory sanogenetic processes are geared up to restore the balance in the body and repair the damage done by a disease. In this situation the body is well prepared for self-healing.

The power of Regimen Therapy is such that often I am reluctant to use any other form of treatment, however non-invasive or safe it may be. For example, when children have frequent colds and coughs, showing signs of a weak immune system, I very often recommend the Regimen Therapy alone without even prescribing any medicine at all other than vitamins or minerals. Children respond so well that they need only simple assistance. They certainly do not need antibiotics for coughs and colds that are viral in nature, since antibiotics have no effect on viruses.

Selecting a treatment

Selecting a particular form of treatment – homoeopathy, acupuncture, Ayurvedic medicine and so on – for a particular ailment is not always as straightforward as I may have made it seem above. There are many overlaps. For example, eczema can be treated by homoeopathy as well as with Ayurvedic remedies. I would normally choose the latter as it is quicker to treat eczema with a selection of herbs than depend on the trial and error method of selecting the appropriate homoeopathic remedy. If the time factor is not important, however, homoeopathy does have its advantages. Herbal medicines may not taste pleasant and may be difficult to prepare (concoct and strain). They may occasionally give undesirable side-effects like loose stools. Homoeopathy on the other hand rarely produces any side-effects. Watch out, however, for the 'healing crisis' when the eczema may suddenly flare up for a brief period. The healing crisis is a very common phenomenon, and its manifestation is a short period of getting worse before you get better. It is a feature of almost all healing to a greater or lesser extent (you cut your finger and it hurts more on the second and third day), but perhaps it is more pronounced in homoeopathy.

Over the years, by carefully observing how different types of treatment produce reactions, I have worked out preferred treatments for various diseases but the individual patient's needs must always be taken into account. For example, if someone is scared of needles then acupuncture is not the best form of treatment because it will create emotional problems. Other factors that need to be considered in choosing the therapies are cost, availability of herbs or remedies, experience of the specialist and individual response to the treatment. Not everyone reacts to treatment in the same way.

I hope this has given you some idea of the range of treatment available out there. Unfortunately you are unlikely to be referred to any of the treatments in this treasure chest by a conventional doctor, who is bound to keep you 'in-house', even if he or she knows, as in liver disorders and eczema, that conventional medicine has no cure while traditional and now integrated medicine has. The term 'general practitioner' is a misnomer to mean general practitioner within conventional medicine. The true GP is the integrated gatekeeper, of whom there are as yet very few.

Chapter 12

ENERGY
Chronic fatigue syndrome

A syndrome is a collection of symptoms, not a disease. Generally a disease is characterised by a cause (agent) and a range of effects (symptoms). Thus tuberculosis is the disease of the lung or other parts of the body that is caused by a bacillus (named after Koch) or bacteria and the symptoms include low-grade fever, toxic weakness and a cough with or without blood and phlegm. This is a disease associated with the toxic effect of the germ. A syndrome is an ailment that is characterised by a group of symptoms and there isn't a definite known cause. Thus premenstrual syndrome (PMS) is characterised by mood fluctuations, water retention, headaches, lethargy and heaviness in the lower abdomen. What its real cause is, is not known, although it is presumed to be due to a lack of the hormone progesterone in the blood as well as pelvic congestion, leading to a decrease in blood supply to the brain. Chronic fatigue syndrome (CFS) illustrates this principle admirably.

Symptoms of CFS

Symptom	System
Fatigue (in 100% of cases)	Energy
Headaches (50%)	Neurological
Depression (50%)	Psychological
Palpitations (20%)	Circulatory
Panic attacks (20%)	Psychological/respiratory
Muscle ache (40%)	Musculo-skeletal
Sleep disturbances (50%)	Psychological
Digestive problems (20%)	Digestive
Short-term memory loss (40%)	Psychological
Lack of concentration (25%)	Psychological
Sore glands (30%)	Immunological
Sore joints (40%)	Musculo-skeletal

Attempts have been made to pinpoint a single cause of CFS but this has been unsuccessful. Since the majority of the symptoms are psychological, there has been a general tendency to categorise the syndrome under psychiatry. Thus this condition received such taunting descriptions as 'yuppie flu' and physicians or psychiatrists used antidepressants to treat it. Coincidentally, patients with CFS using antidepressants often did feel better because these drugs 'masked' the symptoms and boosted their moods. This gave physicians a false confidence about the illness and led them to categorise it as a psychological illness.

Factors contributing to CFS

In my opinion CFS like most diseases and syndromes is a multifactorial condition, where one can confidently say that the symptoms that form part of CFS are caused by different factors acting individually or concurrently.

1

Epstein Barr virus This is the root cause of 25 to 30 per cent of cases of CFS. This virus competes with the body for energy, entering mitochondria (the energy-producing 'power stations' inside cells) and destroying them. Thus the body has a major power failure since mitochondria produce maximum energy in the body. When there is a power failure, every organ and system becomes sluggish and the body becomes 'paralysed' from within. This is the severest form of CFS. The presence of the virus in the tonsils and lymphatic glands causes frequent feverish sensations, swelling of glands, and so on.

Such patients are barely able to move, as muscles, which have an abundance of mitochondria, become inert and lifeless. They ache because the mitochondria are unable to burn glucose properly and so lactic acid accumulates in them.

These patients have all the symptoms of poor physical and mental activity. They suffer very badly and as recovery takes a long time, continue to suffer for years even though viral activity is negligible. This type of CFS is called ME (myalgic encephelomyalitis), which is a misnomer, because it means inflammation of the brain and nerve tissues causing pain in the muscles. This is not the case as it is a name that encompasses a symptom (muscle ache) with a hypothetical condition (inflammation).

2

Neck problems, leading to poor supply of blood to the brain tissue This condition is found in about 60 per cent of cases. American brain mappers have found that part of the brain has poor blood supply in 60 per cent of cases of CFS. Lack of blood flow which results in a poor supply of glucose and oxygen to different parts of the brain, causes chronic fatigue.

Brain cells are very sensitive to lack of oxygen. They can survive for four minutes without oxygen, after which they can die. In CFS there is a reduction in the supply of oxygen, causing the brain cells to suffer from 'power failure' or, in other words, to function with reduced capacity. Brain cells control every part of the body, so if they are not functioning well the body cannot function well either. Memory loss, lack of concentration, fatigue, body ache, headaches, depression and a host of other symptoms can all result.

Two pairs of arteries supply blood to the brain. Each of the carotid arteries supply blood to the face, the skull and the conscious part of the brain (the cortex) – roughly the outer part of the brain, which controls movement, feeling, the psyche, vision, speech and hearing. A stroke along this artery causes paralysis, loss of speech, loss of sensation and so on. A pair of vertebral arteries run through special canals on each side of the cervical spine. Nature has protected this pair of arteries in bony canals because they supply blood to the subconscious brain or brain stem and base. If these arteries fail to supply sufficient blood, the results can include fatigue, headache, emotional problems, poor balance, tinnitus, panic attacks, palpitation, pituitary malfunction (leading to problems with the immune system or hormonal imbalance) and general malaise. See also page 80.

Whiplash injury, producing a range of these symptoms, is a typical example of what can go wrong when the vertebral arteries are slightly compressed due to a misalignment of the cervical spine. The majority of these symptoms are also symptoms of CFS and that is why I presumed that the neck, as well as other neurological, emotional and physical diseases, had something to do with CFS. By correcting the vertebrae of the neck through my technique of massage, manipulation and exercises, I have been able to treat those symptoms. I have been studying the role of the vertebral arteries for over 17 years and my studies will form the subject of a future book.

3

Nutritional deficiency This is another characteristic feature of CFS although whether it is a cause or effect is not known. Many sufferers have deficiency of minerals and often vitamins in the blood when they have CFS. Whether they had it before the symptoms started is not clear, as this is difficult to establish. I have a feeling that sufferers have this problem before the syndrome becomes apparent, or else they would not get a viral attack and feel run down. When suffering from CFS the fatigue is so serious that absorption of minerals, vitamins and other nutrients becomes very sluggish, as do the functions of other organs and systems.

Vitamin and mineral therapy, especially through infusions, have helped many sufferers of CFS, thus indicating a direct link between the two.

4

Yeast and other fungal overgrowth When there is an overgrowth of yeast or candida in the gut, its functions are affected. Bloating, irritable bowel syndrome and other discomforts cause malabsorption of minerals and vitamins, which runs the body down. Moreover, yeast brews alcohol in the gut, utilising various types of carbohydrate present there. Some of these alcohols (such as propanol or butanol) are more toxic than ethanol (found in alcoholic drinks), which is also produced. These toxic alcohols produce deep fatigue. Patients also suffer from bloating, flatulence, poor digestion, occasional diarrhoea and abdominal cramps.

Some sufferers of CFS complain of severe fatigue a couple of hours after a meal. They say their heads become fuzzy and they have extreme fatigue with no power in the body. Such people are usually very intolerant to wine. As much as a sip can cause drowsiness and lethargy. Again, by treating this condition patients become better. Such patients have intolerance to alcohol, especially wine. The alcohol consumes spare oxygen from blood and causes oxygen deficiency in the brain, thus increasing neurological symptoms such as headaches, dizziness and nausea.

Candida overgrowth on the gut lining increases its permeability and certain toxins, which are generally barred from entering the bloodstream, do so, causing chronic fatigue and other neurological/psychological symptoms.

There are many other causes of CFS but they seem to occur less significantly than those mentioned above. These include stress, hormonal malfunction (oestrogen, thyroid), chronic sinusitis, anaemia, low blood pressure, geopathic stress (caused by living near electronic gadgets and high-powered electric cables, etc.) and insomnia.

Treatment

Like all multifactorial diseases, CFS is difficult to treat with one form of therapy. One must take all causative factors and apply treatment to produce a synergistic effect. This is what integrated medicine does best. You must treat the whole body.

The main motive behind all treatments should be to correct the imbalance and give the body a boost of energy. Once you kick-start the body, its own energy-producing system, which is lying dormant, begins to do its job. The body then functions normally on its own.

Regimen Therapy

Regimen therapy is almost essential in CFS as it creates the right background for its healing. Firstly, the patient or sufferer should participate in their own treatment. This is what Regimen Therapy involves. A regime of diet, exercises and massage is essential to create the right amount of energy required to 'kick-start' the process of healing. The 'feel good' factor that Regimen Therapy creates is a good sign of the path to recovery. Without that it is an uphill task – even where the cause is the neck and the correctional therapy there produces an instant spurt of energy as blood flows more freely into the brain. The Regimen Therapy must back up all treatments for any long-term recovery. CFS is a chronic condition and it has to be managed accordingly.

Specialised therapies

1

Massage – manipulative therapy (Dr Ali's technique) Specific spinal treatment, especially to the neck. Since 60 per cent of all sufferers have a neck condition (e.g. pain, stiffness), it has to be treated. Massage the neck and shoulders with Dr Ali's backache oil (see page 164 for the ingredients and preparation method), focusing on the shoulders and the sides of the neck. When massaging the sides of the neck, you may find some tender spots. Massage these areas well till they become less tender. It is best to ask someone else to do it.

Lie on your back. Ask someone to put a small towel around the back of your neck and pull the head away from the torso. Breathe in and out very gently as this is done. This gives the neck a bit of traction.

2

Exercises Do the following exercises described on pages 66–73, which are designed to help back and neck problems: P1, P2, P3, P5, S2, S4, M3, E3, E5 and E6. This set of exercises will mobilise the vertebrae of the neck, and should be done twice a day. Since oxygen deficiency to the brain is a primary cause in many cases of CFS, emphasis should be placed on breathing during the exercise. Besides that, you should walk in the park or in an area where there are trees and fresh air, especially sea air. Walking is a good form of exercise as it is gentle and very effective.

Vigorous exercises are not recommended for people suffering from bad CFS. The body is struggling to generate enough energy to maintain its own metabolism and it is not good to put extra strain on it. In fact most people with CFS have an adverse effect from vigorous exercises. They get very exhausted. You should ration your energy and increase the load on your body very slowly.

3

Nutritional medicine Infusions of vitamins and minerals (B12, Vitamin C, calcium, magnesium, selenium) are very useful in boosting the body's energy to kick-start the process of healing. This treatment is particularly recommended for the post-viral fatigue (ME) type in which sufferers have a devastatingly low level of energy.

The absorption of these vitamins and minerals through the gut is so poor that oral intake does not supply the optimum levels. The severe fatigue blocks the physiological activities that facilitate digestion and absorption. A series of infusions (4–10), done at regular intervals, helps the body to maintain an optimum level of nutrients. This is supplemented by oral vitamins and minerals. The boosted energy facilitates their absorption in the gut, which becomes lazy when the energy level is low. Once the energy level is steady in the body, oral supplements alone can do the job.

4

Acupuncture Many patients have benefited from acupuncture, though for sufferers from post-viral fatigue the results may be slow. If the CFS is connected with stress and neck problems then the release of spasms of the cervical muscles will increase the blood flow to the head. Acupuncture in conjunction with Regimen Therapy does seem to eliminate chronic fatigue.

5

Ayurvedic oil massage Together with Regimen Therapy this form of physical therapy creates the 'feel good' factor which is an essential component of self-healing. The oil massage relaxes the body and mind. Moreover, the herbal oils invigorate the body by improving circulation, removing stiffness and eliminating aches in muscles. Such massages are very useful for convalescing patients and for women after childbirth. The general weakness and fatigue is removed very quickly. Similarly such treatment is useful in CFS.

Prognosis

Since 60 per cent of CFS cases respond to neck adjustment there is a good chance of such cases being improved or even cured. Post-viral chronic fatigue (caused by Epstein Barr virus or others), however, is the most difficult type of CFS to treat. The virus has a devastating effect on the energy-producing system in the body. Repairing and rectifying the system is not an easy task and can take a long time. Young people recover more quickly for obvious reasons.

The fatigue fluctuates in intensity. A person may feel better one day but then have a couple of days of very poor stamina. Such reactions are mostly unpredictable. You have to ration your energy. If you do too much activity in the morning, you must take the afternoon very easily, or else the next day the fatigue will be uncontrollable. This is why people get very depressed. The mind wants to do so many things but the body fails it as physical strength is at a minimum. Sometimes it takes years for the fatigue to go. Sufferers may get used to it by adapting their lifestyle but there is no guarantee that the body will recover fully.

Another type of CFS that responds poorly is the one linked with spinal deformation. Vegetarians with osteoporosis have little chance of making a good recovery. Very few in this category have responded to the integrated medicine approach. The spine shrinks because of osteoporosis and causes permanent obstruction to the blood flow through the vertebral arteries. This produces a deficiency of blood flow to the brain, causing fatigue, dizziness, loss of balance, tinnitus and so on.

I have singled out Western vegetarians, and particularly vegans, because often their protein intake is very erratic as their diet is restricted and does not contain the full range of amino acids needed for the body's own protein synthesis. In cold temperate countries, where there is a lack of sunshine, the synthesis of vitamin D in the skin (its production is facilitated by the sun's rays) is minimal and the only source available is animal protein (meat, eggs, fish). Vitamin D is required for the absorption of calcium in the gut. Taking calcium supplements is useless without vitamin D and without calcium muscles can feel listless and increase the general fatigue.

Energy is necessary for every little function in the body. Lack of it results in 'fatigue', which is only a subjective symptom. It is the tip of the iceberg. A whole series of malfunctions take place, from weakening of the immune, hormonal, circulatory and digestive systems to depression, panic attacks, memory loss and blackouts. Chronic fatigue is a serious condition. Like pain, fever and diarrhoea, which signal to the body that something has gone wrong in the system, fatigue is a symptom that also indicates the failure of a vital system. Energy is the source of life and its deficiency indicates the malfunctioning of the life force, the sanogenetic or healing power. It must therefore be taken seriously.

Chapter 13

THE CIRCULATORY SYSTEM
High blood pressure

The circulatory system feeds and nourishes every other system in the body. Complete failure leads to death, and partial failure affects the whole body, in particular the brain which controls every function of the body, so the effect is both direct and indirect. A common problem affecting the circulatory system is high blood pressure, or hypertension. High blood pressure is usually associated with ageing, but today more and more people aged 40–60 are suffering from it.

Primary and secondary hypertension

About 90 per cent of people with high blood pressure have multifactorial causes, some of which may not be identified. This group of people are said to have primary or essential hypertension. In the remainder of cases the cause is definitely identified and these are classified as secondary hypertension.

There are many causes of primary hypertension which work synergistically or individually. The heart is like a pump and the arteries are like hosepipes (incidentally, veins act passively in the circulatory system). If the pump functions more effectively, the pressure of water/fluid increases. If the hosepipes are squeezed the pressure increases and water comes out with a greater force reaching a further distance.

In secondary hypertension there is always some organic or systemic change that brings about the raised blood pressure. If the lining of the arteries is thickened with plaque formation (cholesterol deposits, fibrous tissue) it is as if the arteries are being squeezed from inside, as opposed to constriction due to spasm of muscles on the outside of the arterial walls. This raises blood pressure.

Similarly, if the kidneys are damaged (due to diabetes, drugs, infection, etc.) certain blood-pressure raising hormones get secreted from the renal tissue (renin-angiotensin reaction) and the result is raised blood pressure.

Normally, if a person runs, the blood pressure rises as the heart rate goes up. After a period of rest, the heart rate and blood pressure return to normal. In a person with mild hypertension the blood pressure returns to normal only after a substantial period of rest. In a person with more severe hypertension the blood pressure only returns to normal after taking some medication. A person can be said to have hypertension as a medical condition if they require treatment to bring the blood pressure down to normal once it has been raised.

Primary hypertension responds to simple medication and can be controlled. Secondary hypertension is difficult to control, as the arteries go through permanent changes or there is a major irreversible change in the body that leads to the high blood pressure. Unless these changes (plaque in arteries, kidney damage) are reversed there is no way of permanently controlling this type of high blood pressure.

Primary hypertension can grow into secondary or permanent hypertension if not controlled properly. The body gives you a chance to counteract the forces that cause primary hypertension before permanent changes take place.

Factors that cause hypertension

1

Genetic factors Hypertension runs in the family so precautions must be taken before the age of 40.

2

Stress Stress hormones raise the heart rate and cause spasm of arterial muscles. Both mechanisms raise blood pressure.

3

Palpitation Resulting from fever, intake of caffeine in large doses, excessive thyroid function, intake of drugs, etc.

4

Kidney malfunction Kidney infection (nephritis), kidney stones, diabetic kidney damage, tumour in kidney, etc. These conditions reduce blood flow to the kidneys and stimulate the secretion of some hormones there that constrict blood vessels and raise blood pressure.

5

Hormonal Intake of oestrogen-based contraceptive pills, steroids (to treat other physical conditions), excessive secretion of hormones from the adrenal glands, etc. can cause blood pressure to rise.

6

Brain or nerve damage and psychic problems (mental disease).

7

Other causes (multifactorial) Primary hypertension (90 per cent of hypertension cases), where the exact cause is not known.

Complications arising from failure to control hypertension

1

Brain haemorrhage Brittle blood vessels of the brain may burst due to very high blood pressure and flood the brain with blood, damaging its tissue.

2

Stroke High blood pressure is the most frequent cause of clot formation in the heart. The heart beats fast and often irregularly, causing a clot to form. This clot travels to the brain and clogs an artery, resulting in a stroke.

3

Retinopathy Small blood vessels in the eye get shrivelled and hardened. These may burst and cause haemorrhage which results in loss of vision. In fact physicians study the state of the smaller blood vessels in order to determine the state of the blood pressure.

4

Kidney damage The small blood vessels of the kidneys may be permanently constricted and cut off the blood supply. This causes the kidneys to shrink and blood pressure to rise permanently.

5

Enlargement of the heart The heart beats fast in people with hypertension. Because it is a muscular organ, the excessive contraction builds up the muscle bulk and this causes enlargement of the left side of the heart. This is a risky complication as permanent heart disease can set in because of poor blood supply to such a bulky heart.

6

Psychological or mood changes People become very irritable.

Development

Hypertension develops in stages:

Stage 1. The blood pressure rises and comes down with or without medication. For example, if one goes through a particularly stressed period, the blood pressure may go up temporarily. With the help of stress management or rest and mild medication, the blood pressure returns to normal.

Stage 2. The blood pressure is continuously raised and medication is essential to bring it down to normal.

Stage 3. Permanent changes take place in the arteries (hardened due to plaque formation) and the blood pressure is brought under control only with great difficulty. Heavy medication is needed.

Treatment

Hypertension is best controlled in the early stages with Regimen Therapy, stress management, or other lifestyle changes. Like all diseases, it is best controlled before it gets chronic. With discipline and effort it can be brought under control in the first two stages of the disease.

Diet

People who suffer from high blood pressure should eat less food. Heavy eating adds to the tension in the body. It is important to keep the body weight under control. Dinner should be very light – salads and soups. Late or heavy dinners are a common factor in weight gain.

In order to control high blood pressure quickly, a **vegetarian diet** is advisable, avoiding meat, poultry and eggs altogether. You can eat fish once a week. Salt is often used in non-vegetarian dishes and moreover they contain animal fat, which is not good for the arteries.

Avoid excess salt, coffee, alcohol, canned products, Chinese food containing monosodium glutamate, fried food, cheese, butter, very spicy food, salt beef, cured meats, red meat, shellfish, sausages, gravy, crisps and chocolates. Sometimes it is advisable to **avoid oils** altogether in cooking – even olive oil, which some say is good for the body. Use spices to flavour the food but add no oil. This will help your weight come down to an optimum level which is good for your body.

It is important to do a **total fast** or a fruit and vegetable soup day once a week. It is best to do it on a Monday as people tend to have large lunches and dinners at the weekend and often overeat. Some people, however, prefer to fast over the weekend. By fasting you avoid salt totally, which is important for treating high blood pressure anyway. Fasting also helps to remove cholesterol from the blood. Regular fasting will help to dissolve some fresh cholesterol deposits on the arteries, and other plaques. Fasting tends to bring down the blood pressure. In fact people with normal blood pressure experience low blood pressure occasionally when fasting.

When fasting, over the course of the day you should drink up to 2 litres of water with a few drops of lemon and honey added. You can also drink Dr Ali's Fasting Tea, which will suppress the appetite to a certain degree. If you feel too hungry, drink a bowl of vegetable soup (without potatoes) at dinner. On a **fruit and soup day** you can eat apples, pears, melon, bananas, grapes, peaches, nectarines, plums and so on, as much as you want, but no citrus fruits. Drink 1½ to 2 litres of water. To make a vegetable soup, boil cabbage, celery, carrots, peas and leeks and add a bit of fresh ginger to it. Drink three to four bowls of this soup throughout the day, without adding any table salt. You may add a bit of magnesium salt (as a replacement for common salt).

Drink carrot and celery juice to **eliminate excess fluid** from the body. This helps to lower the blood pressure. You could also drink nettle tea, which is a mild diuretic. Dr Ali's Water Retention Tea contains useful herbs that eliminate fluid from the body. Drink camomile tea or Dr Ali's Relaxation Tea at bedtime to **reduce stress**.

Massage

A deep-tissue massage every now and then (once a week if your lifestyle is hectic) is very useful in aiding relaxation and therefore helps to lower the blood pressure. Tight muscles in the body increase resistance to the flow of blood and so raise the pressure. Sometimes when there is acute high blood pressure, characterised by sudden headache in the occiput (back of the head), a feeling of agitation and anger, palpitation and tensed muscles, a deep-tissue massage can alleviate the symptoms and lower the blood pressure.

Exercises

The general yoga exercises detailed on pages 64–73, followed by relaxation, are ideal for treating hypertension. The breathing that goes along with the yoga helps to relax the entire body. The heart rate is slowed down and muscle tension is released. This has an important effect on blood pressure. Numerous studies have shown that yoga, relaxation and meditation can lower blood pressure.

The ideal yoga posture for hypertension is 'Shavasana' or 'Dead Man's Posture' (S4). Repeat this exercise morning and evening for 15–20 minutes. The general yoga exercises should be done before the 'Shavasana'.

Exercises like swimming or brisk walking are very good. Competitive games like tennis, squash and golf, where one may perform badly and lose, are not very good for people with high blood pressure. These situations can aggravate the condition and create a foul mood. If you win or play well every time, then the positive emotions that this produces may help to lower blood pressure. Unfortunately such success cannot be guaranteed.

Specific treatments

1

Acupuncture This is a very effective treatment for the early stage of high blood pressure. It releases certain tissue hormones, like endorphins, which relax the entire body. Some acupuncture points like C7 (Heart Meridian) and E36 (Stomach Meridian) can sedate the nervous system and bring the blood pressure down. Sometimes the drop is so sudden that the patient may feel faint or have a sinking feeling with chills, shivers and cold sweat. One has to be vigilant to see that the extreme reaction does not take place. Some acupuncture points can release the spasm of blood vessels (arteries), slow down the heart rate and even increase the urine secretion – all the desired effects of treatment of high blood pressure.

2

Herbal medicine Herbal medicines that lower blood pressure have been in use for hundreds of years. Some 900 years ago, Avicenna wrote a treatise on heart disease and blood disorders describing the use of various herbs in detail. Some Hakims and Vaidas (traditional Unani and Ayurvedic physicians) who taught me gave me various formulations for treatment of hypertension. Here is one I use quite often:

- Sarpgandha – Rauwolfia Serpentina
- Jatamansi – Valeriana
- Shankh Puspi (flowers)
- Gokhru

Rauwolfia Serpentina dilates blood vessels, Valeriana slows the heart rate and dilates arteries, Shankh Puspi is a tranquilliser and Gokhru is a diuretic. These herbs are mixed together in equal proportion. Two tablespoonfuls of the herbs are boiled in 1½ glasses of water for ten minutes and left to cool for an hour or so. Strain and drink the remaining liquid on an empty stomach or in between meals.

Rauwolfia Serpentina, when used as a whole with both the active ingredient as well as antidotes, does not produce the side-effects (depression, suicidal tendencies, etc.) that its derivative resperpine produced when it was openly available as an effective remedy for treatment of hypertension.

3

Homoeopathy This is used for hypertension in the very early stages.

4

Conventional medicines These are divided into the following basic groups:
- drugs slowing down the heart rate (beta-blockers)
- drugs dilating the arterial walls
- drugs that reduce the volume of blood by increasing urine output
- drugs that block blood-pressure-raising hormones in the kidneys
- drugs that block the transmission of impulses to arterial walls, thereby preventing their constriction.

When the blood pressure is very high and complementary and traditional methods of treatment fail to bring about any long-term effect, then conventional medical drugs should be used. Some people are at risk of high blood pressure due to family history, obesity, high-stress jobs and lack of self-discipline. These people are better off taking conventional medical drugs.

Prognosis

It is possible to treat hypertension in the early stage using the integrated medicine approach. As time passes the brain gets conditioned and the high blood pressure becomes permanent. As I said before, as with diabetes, the chances of complications are very high if hypertension is not treated along with a change in lifestyle. The fact that the blood pressure is 'kept under control' with drugs does not guarantee that the complications will not set in. Only a drastic and realistic change in the regimen of diet and exercises can ensure that the control is genuine.

Chapter 14

THE RESPIRATORY SYSTEM
Flu and the common cold

While the circulatory system feeds all the systems of the body, it is itself dependent on the respiratory system for its supply of oxygen and for the elimination of carbon dioxide and waste products. Therefore deterioration of the respiratory system has an immediate debilitating effect on the whole body. This can be seen even in the most common of diseases, such as flu and the common cold.

INFLUENZA

Influenza or flu is a viral fever which is usually seasonal. A change of weather – as in the spring or autumn in temperate countries – generally weakens the body. When the weather is cool one day and hot the next, and when the pattern changes several times during the week, or even over 24 hours, the body is stretched to fine-tune itself to meet the demands of the climate.

In springtime, additional problems arise. It is the end of the season for fruit and vegetables stored from the previous summer. These 'fresh' foods have poor nutrients and, although they look all right, they have poor food value. Where such fruit and vegetables have been in cold storage, they are often in short supply by the end of winter. A shortage of nutrients leaves the body feeling generally run down.

In spring the snow thaws and releases into the atmosphere the germs that it brought down in winter. These weakened germs and viruses seek hosts in whose bodies they can nourish themselves to replenish their species. As if to make matters worse, the viruses which lie dormant to some degree during the winter months suddenly get activated with the first touch of warmth. Sometimes they mutate producing even more virulent types. Then pollens are released into the air causing an additional burden.

As the temperature drops in autumn the weakened viruses seek the comfort of the human body to survive. They sometimes mutate to protect themselves and become extra virulent.

This is why in spring and autumn there are maximum epidemics of viral flu. Epidemiologists get overexcited and microbiologists rush to identify the new strains so that they can make some vaccines or flu jabs to combat the spread of the flu. Whether these vaccines are effective or not is disputable. Vaccinated individuals can get the flu and there is no absolute guarantee.

Viral infection can strike anybody who is run down. It so happens that Christmas time is a very stressful period. While religious festivals all over the world are celebrated with great excitement and enthusiasm, Christmas in Europe can be a time of extra work and worry. Buying presents causes financial stress, while preparing for the dinners (turkeys, special menus, shopping) and children's holidays is a major physical stress. Too many parties and over-indulgence in food and drinks also cause physical stress. Meeting ex-spouses for the sake of family unity causes emotional stress. All this happens at the same time that the body gets very run down and also has to cope with cold weather. It is therefore not uncommon for people to get sick over the Christmas period, though only those who are very run down get flu.

How flu develops

The flu virus lodges itself on the lining of the nose and sinuses as you breathe in the air. The body tries to expel the virus by producing mucus and fluid in the form of a runny nose. This is a full-blown wrestling match between the pathogenetic forces (the virus) and the sanogenetic forces of the body. If the runny nose does not wash the virus off (which it usually does), the virus moves further into the throat and tonsils. This invasion produces the first symptoms of a full-blown flu – fever, sore throat, fatigue, headache (due to the involvement of the sinuses), earache, muscle ache and shivering (due to the toxic effect of the virus).

If the infection is not stopped when it reaches the tonsils, it spreads to the bronchial tract and the lungs. There, too, large amounts of mucus are produced and the body tries to cough up the phlegm. Thus coughing and bronchial symptoms appear.

Viruses are cunning invaders. They enter human cells, stealing their energy and multiplying rapidly. The body's detectives or security guards (the immune system) cannot locate or identify them to make antibodies. External antiviral drugs would have to destroy human cells to get them. Thus viruses go unscathed most of the time.

The fever, which is the main symptom of flu, is the only defensive reaction of the sanogenetic forces that can effectively slow down the activity of the virus. Viral activity and most chemical reactions in the body take place at a certain body temperature, the ideal temperature being 36 °C. If it rises to around 38 °C, these reactions cannot take place and the virus is unable to multiply rapidly. This is how its growth is retarded.

Complications

In the majority of cases the body can easily overcome viral flu, but there can be complications. The most common is secondary infection. Viral flu runs the body down tremendously, thereby giving bacteria in the atmosphere the opportunity to attack it. Moreover, the mucous discharge from the sinuses and the upper respiratory tract is ideal food for the bacteria, so they thrive and multiply rapidly. This makes the bacteria very potent and the infection then spreads to the lungs, causing bronchitis or pneumonia. That is why, when the sputum turns greenish yellow, doctors rush for the antibiotics.

Depending on the virulence of the virus, various organs can be affected, such as the glands, kidneys or brain. These complications can be very serious and it is not unusual to hear of deaths during an epidemic of viral flu. Some strains can cause haemorrhage which can be lethal. Occasionally the virus may attack the brain tissue, causing encephalitis, which is also a serious complication. Glandular fever can linger on for a long time and cause ME or chronic fatigue syndrome.

Treatment

There is a saying that 'If you treat viral flu it will be cured in a week, but if you don't it will get cured in seven days.' Viral flu is a classic example of the sanogenetic forces playing their defensive role. There are no specific antiviral medicines. To fight a virus you have to depend on the body's own immune system. A virus is very cunning. While bacteria and parasites multiply outside the cells, viruses actually penetrate the cells and multiply inside them, destroying those structures that produce antibodies. Thus they are free to do all the damage they can to you, until the body produces interferon, a type of antibody that curbs the activities of the viruses.

The treatment of viral flu is restricted to damage control and helping the physis or sanogenetic forces to gear up their resources to combat the viruses (disease). In fact all diseases should be treated using this model – treat the 'diseased' (the person), not the 'disease' (the virus). Only the body knows the real secret of dealing with a 'cunning' pathogen like a virus, so we need to help it to carry out that function.

Treatment of fever

If the temperature rises up to 39 °C it is OK to use small doses of paracetamol or, better still, cold packs on the forehead or abdomen or air-conditioning on a cool setting. If it touches 40 °C. then paracetamol must be used to bring the temperature down. At such high temperatures the brain functions erratically and the person becomes delirious. The temperature should not be allowed to rise above 40 °C. (or 105 °F) as the body may suffer serious damage, especially nerve cells which are very fragile.

The attitude towards fever or raised body temperature has changed over the past 15 years. Previously it was generally accepted that when you have fever you should cover yourself heavily with blankets and keep warm all the time. Medicine has reversed that view and now advises that the windows be opened, air-conditioning turned on and cold (ice) packs used to force the body to reduce the internal temperature, the aim being to reduce it to below 39 °C, though not necessarily to normal until the virus is overcome. Body temperature is dependent on the outside temperatures of the atmospheric environment. (When you take a hot tub bath your body becomes warmer as its temperature rises.)

Specific treatments

Regimen Therapy consisting of diet, massage, mild relaxation exercises (if possible), particularly S4 (see page 68), and simple remedies are the best cure for flu. Conventional doctors who do not believe in using antibiotics for flu, simply because they do nothing to the virus and are used only as a precaution against secondary bacterial infection, prescribe the following for viral flu:

- bed rest
- plenty of fluids
- vitamins
- paracetamol for fever

The integrated medicine approach to treatment of viral flu consists of the following:

1

Bed rest Viral flu attacks the weakened body and in a full-blown case the body is further affected. It is therefore advisable to rest as much as possible when the flu is at full strength. Rest means total rest in bed with no activities. It is best to sleep as much as possible. This gives the body a chance to rebuild its resources to fight off the virus.

2

Herbal drinks, teas Boil some slices of fresh ginger for five minutes. Strain the water, add honey and a few drops of lemon, and drink this brew every two hours or so. You can add liquorice to the ginger, to reduce inflammation of the throat and lungs. Camomile or rosehip tea is good to drink with honey.

3

Massage Ask somebody to massage your neck, shoulders and spine with some aromatic oils. Ask him or her to concentrate on the neck and shoulder muscles. This part of the body is very tender whenever you are tense and stressed – even before the flu attacks. Massage this area and you will feel much better. Sometimes after a good massage of this area, the temperature will drop instantly. That is probably because the temperature-regulating centre in the brain functions better with the improved blood flow to the brain.

Massage the throat area of the neck with a little oil mixed with eucalyptus and camphor (one teaspoon of base oil to five drops each of eucalyptus and camphor), or use Dr Ali's throat massage oil. While you massage, you'll find several swollen lymph nodes. Massage them well. There will also be sore spots around the muscles and tendons of the floor of the mouth, to be found between the lower jaw and the front of the neck. Massage these well, too. A good massage will relieve the throat pain instantly and you'll be able to swallow better, pain-free.

4

Nose drops Use Dr Ali's sinus oil. Put two drops in each nostril and sniff up. Repeat this twice a day. If you don't have this oil, you can use olive or sesame oil.

5

Supplements
- 500 mg of vitamin C, two or three times per day, and a B-complex will help to boost the system. Sometimes zinc (15 mg) helps to boost the sanogenetic powers against infections.
- Ginseng taken in capsules or tea form is good for flu.
- Chawanprash, an Ayurvedic tonic made up of some two dozen herbs and minerals, is a useful supplement for flu. It has a complete range of herbs that help to energise the body.

6

Homoeopathic remedies are ideal for viral flu. Of all specific treatments perhaps homoeopathic remedies act on the 'diseased' person quickest. If the remedy matches the constitution and the symptoms, the results are quite remarkable and quick. Try Aconite 30 when the fever is very high on the first day, or Gelsemium 30 or Kali Bich 30 – take one tablet three times a day for three days.

Convalescence

This is very important for all acute diseases, especially infections. Most people neglect this period as they consider the absence of symptoms (fever, body ache, cold, sore throat) as the signs of recovery. This is totally wrong. Hippocrates pointed out the importance of a convalescence period in the healing process. In the Greek healing temples, the patients were forced to remain in the convalescence section for a few days after the main symptoms were over. In early Egyptian hospitals patients were actually paid to remain until recovery was complete.

During this period the sanogenetic powers continue to rectify the damage done by the disease to the various organs and systems. Even though the acute symptoms are over, the healing process continues. Take the example of a boil on the skin. The release of pus through the skin (bursting of the boil or abscess) is the moment when all symptoms vanish (pain, throbbing, swelling, fever, etc.) but the inside of the boil is still raw. There are tissue repairs to be taken care of and new cells have to grow to fill the gap. This is what the convalescence period does. It is absolutely foolish to drain the already weakened body even further by not allowing it to rest in the convalescence period.

Post-viral fatigue is the most common outcome of not resting for a couple of days after viral flu leaves the body weak. Chronic fatigue syndrome (see pages 134–141), often resulting from an attack of Epstein Barr virus (ME type), is an example of what can happen if one does not rest after the acute phase of the disease is over.

People are forced to rest after surgery, or a heart attack or a fracture, so why can't we rest after a viral infection, or any acute disease for that matter? We are fortunate that, in most cases, the body copes adequately and does not show any adverse effect, but one should not abuse that power every time. This will ultimately weaken health.

Prognosis

Thanks to our sanogenetic powers, viral flu is cured without much problem. Provided we give the body enough rest and help, the sanogenetic powers will do their job well. It is advisable to take extra care in spring and autumn by following the Regimen Therapy as a precautionary measure even though you might feel apparently 'fit'. You can do a self assessment (pages 120–121) to check your state of health.

THE COMMON COLD

They say that medical science has made such great technological advances that a surgeon in London can remove the gall bladder of a patient in Sydney through telemedicine. Yet it has not been able to find a cure for the common cold. Conventional medicine knows it is some sort of a virus so all one can do is hope for the body to heal on its own, as in flu. As mentioned earlier, the curing of the common cold on its own is a clear example of the sanogenetic powers or healing force of the body. The seven-day rule applies to this too. There is nothing a doctor can do to treat the virus, but the body has its own tactics for dealing with it.

The most important fact behind a common cold is that the body is always run down before it catches a cold. When you catch a 'chill' by exposure to cold air, air-conditioning, getting wet (especially in the head) and so on, the body's energy is wasted in warming it up. As a result of that there is an acute loss of the 'inner heat' and the body gears up its resources to compensate for that. This makes the immune system vulnerable. Opportunistic viruses, present in abundance in the air, then try to enter the body through the nasal passage where they begin to thrive.

In a defensive reaction the mucus in the nose increases to 'wash' the virus out. The wrestling match between the pathogenetic force (the virus) and the sanogenetic powers (shown in the mucus discharge) is in full swing. In most cases the body wins and the virus is eliminated. If the body loses, the virus penetrates deeper into the throat, sinuses and lungs, causing inflammation of these organs. There is, however, no fever as in flu.

Treatment

The most sensible thing to do in this case is to help the body to eliminate the virus. Stopping the cold with antihistamine or nasal sprays that constrict blood vessels to stop fluid filtering through them, is not a good idea, however convenient it might be for the patient. Here are some tips on treatment.

Diet

Avoid the following:
- cold water or chilled drinks (warm drinks like herbal tea or warm water help to eliminate the cold)
- dairy products – they increase mucus production
- fungal products – mushrooms and cheese.

Try the following:

- **ginger and black pepper tea** Boil a few slices of fresh ginger with a pinch of black pepper for four to five minutes. Add a few drops of lemon and drink with a little organic honey.
- **anti-cold soup** Chop onion, ginger, leek, a bit of garlic and some potatoes. Boil these in water for 20–25 minutes. Add a bit of mustard paste, black pepper, salt and a few drops of lemon. (You can also use fresh chicken stock or bone marrow stock to prepare this soup.) Drink it twice a day. After drinking this soup your body will warm up and you might sweat in the forehead.
- **brandy with honey** A teaspoonful of brandy with honey in a cup of warm water at bedtime is useful.

Other treatments

1 **Nose drops** Sniff equal quantities of mustard and pure sesame oils or use Dr Ali's sinus oil. Put one drop of this mixture of oils in each nostril and sniff up. Do this twice a day. Mustard has a powerful antibacterial property and possibly some antiviral property.
2 **Nasal douche** Take a Neti pot (used in yoga) or use a tea pot. Fill it with luke-warm water and add half a teaspoonful (to a glass) of table salt. Tilt your head to the left, open your mouth wide and breathe through your mouth. Insert the spout into the right nostril and pour the saline water into the nostril. Breathe only through the mouth, and if you do so the water will come out of the left nostril. Repeat the same by tilting your head to the right and pouring the water into the left nostril. This procedure will help the body to wash away the virus. Make sure you dry your nostrils with cleansing breath (see page 64).
3 **High dose of vitamin C** 500 mg, two to three times a day for five days.
4 **Homoeopathic remedies** See a physician or try Ferrum Phos, Aconite 30 or Gelsemium 30. Take one tablet three times a day for three days.

Prognosis

If the cold is treated as soon as it starts (with sneezing or a running nose) then the secondary complications (sinusitis, pharyngitis) do not set in. It is good to have a cold every now and then. It gives you a chance to pay attention to your body.

Chapter 15

THE MUSCULO-SKELETAL SYSTEM
Backache

Of all the musculo-skeletal diseases, backache is the most common and extensively studied complaint of modern urban society. It has many causes. Probably 80 per cent of people with backache have a problem related to the discs. Backache can also be caused by arthritis of the vertebral joints, osteoporosis, growing pains, or referred pain caused by kidney problems, gynaecological problems, or problems of the digestive system. I have been treating people with backache for the past 20 years and have tried to analyse the condition very closely. I use massage and yoga therapy. By touching and feeling the muscles, joints and bones, I have acquired a lot of information about the conditions that lead to backache and have been able to see a pattern in the various types that occur.

In this chapter I am going to focus on disc-related backache with a brief look at backache caused by other factors on pages 168–169.

Before I go on to describe treatments, let me briefly explain my theory about the spine and how backache originates. Without this explanation one cannot see the logic behind my treatment.

Evolution of the human spine

Homo erectus, the first species of human, walked erect, probably to get a better view and reach out for things, and developed an unusual spine. How does the human spine function?

The spine is at the back of the body and the organs are in front of it. Except for the spinal muscles and the skin, there is nothing behind the spine. Liver, lungs, heart, spleen, intestines, uterus, bladder and so on are all in front of the spine. This is where the body's engineering has gone apparently wrong, as if the creator had made a mistake. Normally, weight is distributed around a central axis, like the trunk of a tree with branches growing in different directions. In the animal kingdom, the spine acts as a horizontal 'pole' supported at either end by two vertical stands (fore and hind legs). From this 'pole' hang the thoracic and abdominal organs. It is a perfect piece of structural engineering. But in human beings all the weight is at the front.

The trouble is that humans were not designed to stand erect and walk. The spine was designed for a horizontal position, but it is made to stand erect. As a result the largest vertebrae are at the bottom and not round the shoulder region as in four-legged animals. The spine has a tendency to tilt forward, because of the weight of the organs and the back muscles have to contract to pull the spine up like a pulley. The body has a tendency to stoop or lean forward while the back muscles try to prevent it. This happens every time we stand or sit, putting continuous strain on the ligaments and muscles of the spine. When one snoozes in an erect position, the head drops forward with a jerk. (See diagrams a, b, c overleaf.)

Abdominal muscles play an indirect minimal role in maintaining the erect posture and thus preventing backache. Some people are obsessed with strengthening the abdominals for curing backache. These muscles only help to 'tuck' the tummy bulge in to keep the internal organs in position, so that the centre of gravity is where it should be, at the base of the spine. This reduces the load on spinal muscles and aids their pulley action. Thus abdominals play an important secondary role only when the tummy bulges.

Role of spinal muscles

A skeleton cannot stay erect without the active participation of muscles. In the erect position, human spinal muscles must extend, or else the body's weight could not be supported vertically. The pulley system alone could be strong enough to pull the body upright against the weight of the organs, which tend to tilt it forward. Only an upward force can make this possible. This force can be created only by muscles with powers to extend. I call this the anti-gravitational force. This force counteracts the weight of the body (gravitational force) as well as extending the spine to maintain an erect posture. Thus the total anti-gravitational force must equal the body's weight. In addition it must keep the spine erect with a force that stretches the spine upwards. (See diagram d.)

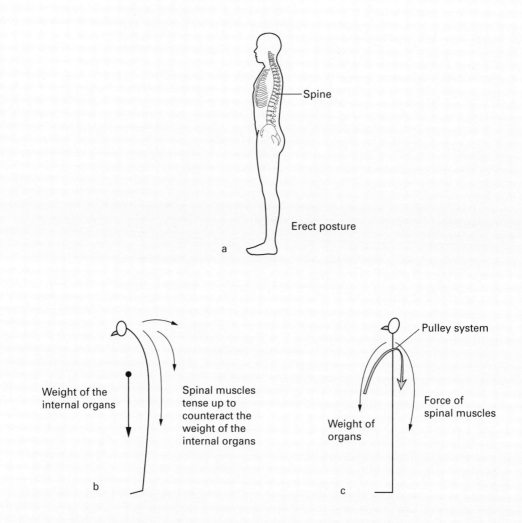

Spine

Erect posture

a

Weight of the internal organs

Spinal muscles tense up to counteract the weight of the internal organs

b

Pulley system

Weight of organs

Force of spinal muscles

c

In a paralysed person or a dead body, the anti-gravitational force is absent. The body feels heavier hence the expression 'deadweight'. The opposite can also happen. Ballerinas and exponents of martial arts train themselves to be 'weightless' so that they can 'fly in the air'. In a deeper state of meditation, the spine is stretched upwards to neutralise forces of gravity and as a result of that many people have experienced 'levitation'. The person can spring up and often jump like a frog for a metre or so. The upward thrust is helped with a slight upward push of knees, thighs and seat muscles, and possibly by sudden extension of all the spinal muscles. This slight propulsion gives the body the lift, a dynamic process in which the bones play no active part.

Thus muscles and not the vertebrae or bones play the main role in maintaining the posture. The vertebrae provide the necessary surfaces to which muscles are attached and together they provide the strength and power that is required in maintaining the erect posture.

Role of discs

Orthopaedic surgeons and physicians who deal with backache are obsessed with discs as the primary cause of backache. In a typical situation, they say a disc bulges or herniates, touching nerves emerging out of the spine and, by scratching or compressing them, produces backache and other neurological symptoms. The disc compression in my view is an effect and not a cause. The main reason why discs compress is the weakening of the anti-gravitational force (sloppiness of the spinal muscles). When the upward thrust is weakened, the downward gravitational force is relatively increased. This force compresses the disc. The anti-gravitational force, when in full strength, should keep the discs inflated. The factors that cause discs to be compressed and finally degenerate are:

- **weakening of the anti-gravitational force** by fatigue, stress, illness, lack of exercise, nutritional imbalance, insomnia
- **increase in body weight**, especially sudden weight gain
- **trauma**, (e.g. road accident)
- **ageing**
- **bad posture** (poor extension of the spine).

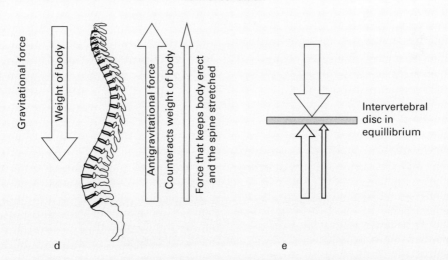

Like speech or breathing the body's erect posture is mostly controlled by the subconscious (involuntary) part of the brain. It can also be controlled voluntarily, or by the conscious brain. The Alexander Technique teaches you to maintain optimum posture by 'training the brain'. Thus the posture is good when you are healthy and mentally relaxed. If you are stressed or tense, the muscles will automatically tighten up. When spinal muscles tighten up or contract with stress, they compress the discs, since the vertebrae are drawn nearer to each other with contraction.

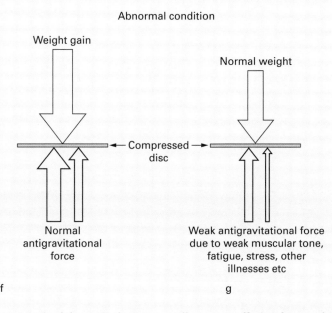

Abnormal condition

Weight gain

Normal weight

← Compressed →
disc

Normal
antigravitational
force

Weak antigravitational force
due to weak muscular tone,
fatigue, stress, other
illnesses etc

f   g

When you are tired, haven't slept very well, or are suffering from a chronic disease or simply poorly in health, your muscles lack tone. You feel lazy and inactive. This reduces the power of the anti-gravitational force and thus the discs get compressed and may finally degenerate (see diagram above).

Trauma can weaken the muscles and ligaments. It can also directly affect the vertebrae and cause rupture of the discs.

The most interesting thing is that since erect posture is maintained by the involuntary forces, voluntary exercises, especially vigorous ones, may not prevent disc compression and relieve backache. Thus exercise such as weightlifting, aerobics or running may not help a disc problem as they rely on voluntary contraction of spinal muscles. Swimming and yoga, on the other hand, are extremely useful in treatment and prevention of backache, as they rely heavily on the subconscious mind. People who are calm and relaxed or enjoy well-being rarely have backache. Athletes who are very stressed, however, may be very strong physically but often suffer from a bad back. Thus it is well-being and health which determine the state of the back. Bad posture, poor nutrition, excess weight and repetitive strain play some role in the genesis of backaches, but there are other hidden factors that play a much bigger role.

DISC-RELATED BACKACHE

This is by far the commonest form of backache and it can be acute, when due to a sudden movement there is a slight 'snap' followed by an excruciating pain. This is often referred to as 'slipped disc'. Due to the weakening of the muscles and ligaments that bind the vertebrae of the spine together, the vertebrae can easily shift or become misaligned. As a result of this slight shift, they become more vulnerable to a greater displacement under strain or sudden movement. Once displaced, the joints that connect vertebrae are dislocated and the disc is unevenly compressed. This pressure on the disc causes it to bulge at its weakest point and this protrusion impinges on the of nerve roots. That is the origin of the excruciating pain.

When the spine is in a healthy condition an acute prolapse of a disc is only possible if there is a fall or trauma such as an accident. Sudden movement alone will not cause it. You don't see Pete Sampras slip a disc, for all his bending and picking up tennis balls. When a slipped disc occurs after lifting or bending, it is usually because the disc is already compressed or weakened by the factors mentioned on page 161. Moreover, the muscles and ligaments that bind these vertebrae together are weakened or strained long before the episode takes place. The sudden movement is just something that triggers the bulge or aggravates it.

Chronic wear and tear of an inadaquately supported disc can cause gradual degeneration. In this case the blood supply to the disc is cut off due to compression and the soft material withers away, slowly being replaced by bone tissue. Excess body weight and lack of exercise can promote and accelerate the degeneration. Such a disc degeneration or prolapse can happen anywhere in the spine but the most frequent location is in the lumbar region and the lower part of the neck, where the wear and tear is greater. Thus tingling or numbness down the arm into the fingers and sciatica in the leg, caused by pressure on the nerves, are more common than such disorders in other areas of the body.

Nutritional problems can also cause disc degeneration. When there is an imbalance of nutrition due either to poor intake or poor absorption in the gut, the body gets generally run down and the anti-gravitational force is weakened. Moreover, nutritional imbalance can cause changes in joints and bones.

Treatment of disc-related backache

I have derived a range of treatment for backache, based on my observation of the various structures and symptoms. Once again an integrated approach seems to be the best solution.

Diet

An optimum weight has to be maintained to keep the discs intact. As a rough guide take your height in centimetres and subtract 100 to get your optimum weight in kilograms. Thus if you are 160 centimetres tall, your ideal weight should be 60 kg (see page 107 for a more accurate method of working out your ideal weight).

If your weight increases above the optimum level the muscle power and especially the anti-gravitational force should be increased through various exercises to counteract the effect or else the discs will come under pressure. You must maintain a balance between your weight and the muscle tone in the spine. If you follow the diet recommended on pages 50–54 you should be able to maintain an optimum weight.

Massage therapy

There is no better treatment for muscles than massage and moreover it gives comfort to and relaxes the entire body. When you have a backache the muscles tense up, either due to the compression of the nerves in the affected segment of the spine or due to accumulation of lactic acid. Normally glucose (energy) molecules react with oxygen in the blood to form carbon dioxide and water, which are naturally eliminated. When muscles overwork, however, the supply of oxygen cannot meet the demand and some glucose molecules are only converted to lactic acid, a product requiring less oxygen. Massage brings in more blood and therefore more oxygen, allowing lactic acid to be converted to the end products (carbon dioxide and water).

Accumulation of lactic acid causes muscle spasms and hardened 'knots' form in them. These 'knots' interfere with the transmission of power along muscles by causing interruptions in the pathway. They make muscles inert or less effective. Moreover these knots are sites of great pain and discomfort. If they are not released, then fibrous tissue may grow into them and immobilise them. The hardened or fibrosed knots become permanent sites of pain in the spine. This condition is often referred to as fibromyalgia (*fibro* – fibrous tissue; *myalgia* – pain in muscles or myos). The sooner such knots are flattened out through massage, the better it is for the spine.

> **Use Dr Ali's backache oil for massage. This oil consists of the following ingredients (use a teaspoon as the basic measure):**
>
> 2 parts mustard oil – to warm the muscles and improve blood flow
> ½ part camphor oil – to soothe the muscles
> ½ part clove oil – as painkiller
> 4 parts sesame oil – to nourish (rich in Vitamin D)
> 1 part black cumin seed oil – as anti-inflammatory remedy

The oil is massaged into the spinal muscles, which are easily identified along the length of the spine. it is important to massage along the entire spine, not just where the pain is, as the spinal muscles, not all of which run along the entire length of the spine, act as one. Together they create the anti-gravitational force. Rubbing only the sore area will remove the immediate pain but will not help to treat the decompression of discs, the root problem causing such pain.

The neck muscles end up in tendons which are attached to the base of the skull. These tendons are the continuation of the muscles and play an equal role in the maintenance of tone and power in them. These tendons, which are usually very sore, have to be massaged until they ease up. Similarly the lumbar and lower back muscles end up in a cord of strong tendons which are attached to the sacrum, the last part of the vertebral column. If you run your thumb or finger down the muscles of the lower back, you'll feel that, at the end, the soft muscles transform into cord-like tendons. These tendons are usually very tender whenever there is a lower back problem. By massaging the tendons, you bring more blood to them. Tendons have a poor blood supply, which is why they are white in colour and they heal so slowly when they become inflamed. Massage helps them to recover more quickly.

The gluteal or seat muscles and the hamstrings (behind the thighs) also need massage. When these muscles tense up, for example after sitting for a long time, they affect the lower back. One must also remember that these seat muscles and hamstrings play a role in preventing the forward stoop of the body by pulling the spine back. They too get fatigued and strained while maintaining the erect posture, and especially when in motion. These are muscles that help to bring the body back to its erect position by acting as 'pulleys'. Imagine a game of tennis or squash when the player bends low to pick up the ball and then springs back to the erect position. It is the spinal, gluteal muscles and hamstrings (even the calves) that make such movements possible by working synergistically.

Exercises

The entire spine has to be exercised to cure and prevent backache. The following exercises which are described on pages 66–73, are designed to work on muscles, tendons and joints – all the parts that are directly involved in backache: P1, P2, P3, P5, S2, S4, M3, E3, E5 and E6.

Posture

Maintaining the correct posture is essential in keeping the spine aligned. The majority of abnormalities in the discs and joints of the spine arise from bad posture which causes abnormal tension in certain groups of muscles, ultimately weakening them. The **Alexander Technique** is an excellent method of posture therapy.

While sitting or standing you should feel as if your head is being held upright by an upward stretching force. To experience this, push your shoulders back to a comfortable position (i.e. not experiencing any discomfort) and raise your chin up until you feel the release of tension in the neck muscles at the back. At this point, allow your neck to float upwards a bit until the neck and shoulder muscles are free of any strain or tension. Practice this several times a day whenever you are conscious of your posture. After a while it will become a habit. Subconsciously you will be able to maintain this posture.

Manipulation

Manipulation by osteopathy, chiropractic and other techniques, when done at an appropriate time, is extremely beneficial. Sometimes the results are instantaneous, as the treatment removes the immediate cause of the pain (such as misalignment of vertebrae causing impingement on the nerves).

An experienced therapist will take only a few sessions to resolve the problem and will rely on the body's own ability to maintain the status quo in the back. He or she will know that frequent manipulation ultimately makes the back lazy. Always look for an experienced osteopath or chiropractor. A combination of exercises, massage and gentle but infrequent manipulation of the back should take care of backache. Therapists who insist on manipulation only, and do not recommend any exercises to back up the therapy, are probably not interested in a long-term cure and merely want to keep the symptoms under control. Some patients love this kind of approach as it is an easy way out of pain and they do not have to lose weight, do exercises and manage stress with a lifestyle change.

Acupuncture

This is another excellent therapy for acute and chronic backache. Sometimes the backache is so acute that massages, manipulation and exercises become impossible to carry out. The patient may be in such a vicious circle of pain and fear of more pain that acupuncture is the only treatment that can break the cycle. In the hands of an experienced acupuncturist, the therapeutic effect is as powerful as a block with anti-inflammatory drugs injected directly into the muscle. In chronic backache, especially in the elderly, it becomes an essential therapy in conjunction with massage and exercises, especially when spinal manipulation is contraindicated.

Acupuncture not only removes muscular spasm and pain, but acts as an anti-inflammatory procedure. It should not be taken as an easy way out for 'lazy' people. Exercises must be done to consolidate the effect of relief of pain and discomfort.

Ayurvedic oil massage

Hot medicated oils are massaged into the back and rubbed into the muscles. This is done for about ten days in a row. The anti-inflammatory properties of the oil are particularly beneficial for backache that originates from muscles, such as **Polymyalgia rheumatica** (rheumatic muscle ache) an inflammatory disease of the muscles, mostly affecting the spine, which is a very painful condition. Backache caused by **arthritis** can also be treated by this method.

Back surgery

Back surgery is sometimes necessary, but it should only be considered when other avenues have been tried and failed. Surgery should be postponed as long as possible in most cases, but in some the damage to the disc or the nerves they impinge on may be so great that it becomes unavoidable. Surgery may be required in the following situations:

1

Foot drop The compression of the nerve roots in the lumbar spine causes nerve damage making the foot drop. It cannot be lifted up as it is paralysed. Surgery can remove the compression and the hope is that the foot will regain its power as a result. The sooner the surgery is done, the better chance there is of recovery.

2

Burning, tingling or numbness in the sciatic region Persistent numbness is also caused by nerve damage. Where the bladder and bowel is involved, urgent treatment is needed.

3

Rupture of the disc after a trauma In these situations the compression or fracture may be irreversible. The pain and the loss of muscle tone should be the main considerations in deciding whether to operate.

4

Severe pain leading to disability When a patient's life is restricted to bed rest due to severe pain and he is unable to carry out any function, then surgery should be considered.

5

Loss of power in the hands, severe pain in the arm and numbness in the fingers which is persistant. When conservative treatment fails in these situations then surgery is recommended.

Before you go for surgery, prepare your spinal muscles with massages and exercises, for it will take weeks before you can do anything with your back. The muscles might atrophy.

Prognosis

Backache can be debilitating, although people react differently depending on their pain threshold. Some people are so impatient that after suffering for a few months they go for surgery. Some neurosurgeons and orthopaedic surgeons are 'knife' hungry. They do not believe in any conservative treatment, although the acceptance of osteopathy and chiropractic by conventional medicine in recent times has changed the views of many surgeons. Many of them suffer from backaches themselves and are fully aware of the complications of surgery. They seek conservative therapy first.

Back surgery is not without complications. As the technology has advanced, and with the introduction of keyhole surgery, minimal damage is done to the spine. A new technology is being developed to 'cement' the disc area with a chemical. This means the surgery can be done with the help of a needle and the patient does not need to be opened. Such surgeries will revolutionise the treatment of complicated backache.

Prevention of backache by maintaining optimum weight, with a healthy lifestyle using Regimen Therapy, is the best solution. Sleep is also a contributory factor. The only time muscles relax fully is when you go into a deep sleep. If you have a disturbed or interrupted sleep the muscles get fatigued. This leads to chronic backache. You should sleep as much as possible to prevent backache.

Treatment for backache resulting from other causes

Osteoporosis-related backache

- **Diet** Make sure your diet is high in protein – fish, chicken, cottage cheese, almonds (soaked for 24 hours), tofu, etc.
- **Treat** constipation or irritable bowel syndrome, if affected (see pages 211–213 for advice on diet).
- **Coral calcium** This calcium supplement is imported from Japan (available from the Integrated Medical Centre). Soak a couple of sachets in a litre of water and drink over the course of a day. The dissolved calcium is easily absorbed by the gut.
- **Massage** Use Dr Ali's osteo oil, which is made up of equal parts of mustard, avocado and sesame oil. Use two teaspoons of each oil per application and massage well all over the body, until it is fully absorbed. Do not bathe for 6–8 hours after application, as this gives the body a chance to absorb Vitamin D from the oils. Mustard oil acts as an irritant, drawing blood into the muscles, ligaments and bones, thus bringing extra supplies of calcium to them.

Osteoarthritis

Osteoarthritis is a common cause of backache, although it affects not only the spine but also the weight-bearing joints of the hips, knees, ankles, toes, shoulders, elbows and hands.

Treatment

- **Diet** Avoid dairy products, sugar, coffee, citrus fruits and excess fat. It is best to avoid red meat altogether. Include in your diet fenugreek – as a vegetable, cooked in a little oil, ginger, sesame seeds or oil, olives, soaked almonds and carrots. Chop one or two garlic cloves and swallow them with a little water each day.
- **Anti-inflammatory treatments** Take 1/2 teaspoon of powdered ginger with a little honey, or try gum arabica or guggal in tablet or capsule form.
- **Massage** of the affected joints with Ayurvedic oils is very useful. Try Mahanarayan oil or Dhawanthari oil, or my own anti-arthritic oil. To make this up, mix two parts of sesame oil with two parts of mustard oil, one part of olive oil, one part of clove oil and one part of turpentine oil. Massage into the joints and leave overnight.

Arthritis-related backache

- Follow the diet and treatment suggested for arthritis (page 166).

Growing pains

Between the ages of about 10 and 20 rapid growth can cause back pain. The bones of the spine grow rapidly and the muscles cannot keep pace. The tendons stretch like the string of a bow and get inflamed causing excruciating pain.

- **Massage** the spinal muscles, concentrating on the nape of the neck and the base of the spine where such tendons hurt most. Use Dr Ali's back massage oil (see page 164).
- Do the **yoga exercises** recommended for backache: P1, P2, P3, P5, S2, S4, M3, E3, E5 and E6 (pages 66–73).

16

THE NEUROLOGICAL SYSTEM
Headaches and migraine

The nervous system is probably the most complex and miraculous system in the body, including as it does the brain. It is also the least understood. When it goes wrong it generally affects the whole body and can be devastating, as in migraine, and it may even manifest itself in no more than a mild headache. Problems affecting the nervous system are generally multifactorial, giving integrated medicine a big advantage.

HEADACHES

Few people can claim never to have had any headache, even a brief one. Most people take it as a passing symptom but for some it is a matter of concern. Like all forms of pain in the body, a headache is a signal or warning that something is wrong in the head or another part of the body. It tells you to pay attention to your body. In some cases it stops you completely and cries out for total rest. Headache itself is not a disease but a symptom of an abnormal condition. Similarly, fatigue, pain, fever, diarrhoea, cough, sneezing, rashes on the skin, or a runny nose are all symptoms of disease but are not themselves diseases.

Causes of headaches

Headaches can affect different areas of the skull, and the location of the pain can give clues to its cause.

1

General headaches (all over) These can be caused by low or high blood pressure, anaemia, increased pressure of the brain fluid, allergy, toxins (chemicals like wet paint), low blood sugar, high blood sugar, dehydration, brain tumour, meningitis, low oxygen pressure (altitude sickness), arteritis (inflammation of arteries in the brain or head), low thyroid or high thyroid function, low estrogen levels etc.

2

Frontal headache (forehead) These can be caused by tension or stress (frontal lobe of the brain), sinus problems, weak eyesight, photosensitivity (sensitivity to bright light), susceptibility to radiation (x-rays, electronic gadgets).

3

Unilateral headache Pain on only the right or only the left side can be caused by migraine, occlusion of the vertebral artery, inflammation of the joint of the jaw (located in front of the ear), toothache, trauma (bump, hurt), whiplash, tightening or injury of the biting muscles, trigeminal neuralgia etc.

4

Headache in the occiput (back of the skull) Pain here can result from injury or tension of neck muscles, high blood pressure (when it is not too high) in the initial phase, dislocation of joints of the cervical spine, computer strain, torticollis (twisted neck due to sleeping badly in an awkward position or due to drug reaction), neuralgia of the occiputal nerve.

5

Pain at the top of the head Headaches here can indicate high or low blood pressure, and meningitis. If you have other symptoms associated with meningitis such as a stiff neck and a suspicious rash, you need to seek urgent medical attention.

Thus you can see how many different causes of headaches there are. If one were to classify them according to their causes one would come up with the following groups: circulatory (e.g. high blood pressure), trauma (whiplash), infection (meningitis), allergy (sinusitis, wet paint), growth or tumour (cyst in the brain or tumour), deficiency (anaemia, low blood sugar), neuralgia (trigeminal) and hormonal (thyroid).

Headache is a symptom that can happen when the blood pressure is high or low, the blood sugar level is high or low, or the atmospheric pressure is high or low. It seems that what really matters is the irritation of the membranes of the brain, by chemicals or increased pressure or inflammation where the pain receptors are. As I mentioned before the brain tissue itself has no pain receptors, although it is concentrated with nerve cells and nerve fibres. Thus a tumour may silently grow within the brain tissue, causing neurological symptoms in various parts of the body (impaired gait, tingling, loss of muscle power, etc.) and not be noticed until headaches start due to increased pressure of brain fluid. Unless it is so large as to block fluid circulation, which may irritate the meningeal (brain membrane) pain receptors, it will not cause any pain in the head. A vigilant doctor may ask for a scan and be surprised to discover a brain tumour.

There are nerve endings on the arteries in the base of the brain. Inflammation or pressure on them may also trigger pain in the head.

Some headaches are caused by general problems in the body. They are usually toxic. In fevers, where sinuses are not involved, there is always a headache. Chronic constipation causes irritation of the mucus membrane of the sinuses because the body secretes mucus to eliminate toxins. The thick fluid accumulates in the sinuses and causes the pressure in them to increase. Chronic fatigue, insomnia and depression cause a low-grade headache, mainly due to poor oxygen or glucose supply to the brain membranes.

Most headaches are one-sided and the rest are general. My hypothesis is that circulatory headaches are one-sided – migraine, headaches caused by temporal arteritis, vertebral artery compression or occlusion on one side, and so on. Other unilateral headaches are caused by inflammation of the jaw joint and neuralgias.

Identifying the cause of a headache

As there are so many causes of headaches you must carry out some simple checks, like the preliminary questioning by a detective.

1

If the headache is one-sided, severe, lasts over a day, causes nausea and vomiting, or hypersensitivity to light and sound, appears before periods in a monthly cycle, or appears in certain cycles during the month, the chances are that it is migraine. See pages 176–181 for more information about this problem.

2

If the headache is one-sided, throbbing though not accompanied by nausea or vomiting, but accompanied by extreme tenderness on one side of the neck, then it is caused by vertebral arterial occlusion. These headaches are aggravated by fatigue, exertion, jet lag, cervical spondylitis (neck pain), computer overuse or whiplash injury. These headaches can be frequent but follow no cyclical pattern. Note that this type of headache can also be the result of temporal arteritis (inflammation of the temporal artery) which will need urgent treatment.

3

If the headache is general or all over the head, then ask yourself a few questions like: is there any link with hunger? Low blood pressure? High blood pressure? Allergies? Hormonal problems like low thyroid function? If you can't identify any definite cause, ask your doctor to carry out some investigations.

4

If there is a frontal (forehead) headache, ask yourself these questions: Are you constipated? Are you stressed? Do you have hypersensitivity when looking into bright light? Is there any mucus discharge from the sinuses down into the throat? If you think you have sinus headache, press the two points at the inner end of the eyebrows with your fingers. If these points are sensitive, the headache you have is from congestion in the sinuses. You should also check your eyesight.

5

Press the jaw joint in front of the ear. If it is painful especially when you open your mouth, the joint is inflamed. Pain may be spreading from this joint to one side of the head.

Most of the headaches fall into the above categories and diseases like brain tumour, aneurisms (bulbous swellings of arteries) and brain haemorrhage are not so common. In any case, if the simple treatments recommended below help to eliminate the headache, the chances are that what you diagnosed was correct.

Certain types of headache, like those that come on while coughing, during sexual intercourse, walking upstairs and so on (known as 'exertional headaches'), are easy to diagnose. These are easily triggered off by misalignment of the vertebrae of the neck, which press on the vertebral artery during movement or exertion. The restricted blood flow through this artery causes the headache.

Treatment

If the cause is known then treat it and the symptom (headache) will be cured. Unfortunately it is sometimes quite difficult to establish the cause. General treatments like Regimen Therapy can improve the well-being of a person and thereby treat headaches, together with other underlying symptoms.

Diet

If allergy or constipation are causing the headache, diet is very important. Avoid coffee, cheese, mushrooms, milk, MSG (Chinese food flavouring), excess salt, very spicy food, citric juices, yeast products, fried food, shellfish, and excess alcohol (you should especially avoid beer, wine, bitter and champagne).

Massage

Massage is very important for curing acute and chronic headaches. Ask somebody to massage your neck and shoulders with some oil, focusing on the sides of the neck and the back of the head. For acute headache a massage of this area for 10–15 minutes with a slight traction (pulling of the head away from the shoulders) should release the headache. Massage the temples and the jaw muscles to release tension in them.

If sinuses are causing the headache, put two drops of Dr Ali's sinus oil drops into each nostril and sniff up. (Alternatively, use organic sesame oil.) Massage the two pressure points at the end of the inner side of the eyebrows.

If inflammation of the jaw joint is responsible for the headache, massage the affected joint in front of the ear with Tiger Balm or Dr Ali's arthritis oil for a few minutes. Open the jaws a few times as you massage. If it is still very sore and feels swollen (due to fluids in the joint), use a hot salt poultice. Heat a cup of salt in a pan for five minutes. Pour hot salt into a handkerchief, tie it up to make a poultice bulb and hold it against the painful area.

Exercises

Yoga exercises are an excellent remedy for acute and chronic headaches, particularly the following, detailed on pages 64–73: Cleansing Breath B 1–6, Cobra (half) P2, Turtle M2, Semi-bridge S3, Neck Twist E6, Self-traction P3, Head Roll E5.

Acute headache

This is an uncomfortable symptom and it ought to be treated immediately. The best thing to do is to assess the underlying cause of the headache and treat it. Neck and shoulder massage, as I mentioned earlier, can release the headache immediately by allowing more blood (carrying oxygen and glucose) into the brain. If there is an opportunity to do the set of 12 exercises recommended above before massage, you should feel even better.

Medicines and speciality treatment

1

Ginger and camomile tea

2

Acupuncture relieves various types of headaches quickly.

3

Osteopathic or chiropractic manipulation readjusts the misaligned vertebrae in the cervical spine and releases the headache.

4

Cranial osteopathy – this gentle treatment of the cranium improves the circulation of cerebro-spinal fluid to the brain.

5

Conventional medicines like aspirin and paracetamol should be used if the above methods fail to release the headache. Preference should always be given to the Regimen Therapy, acupuncture and manipulative therapy because they stand a better chance of getting at the cause.

Prognosis

Headaches are annoying symptoms. They return every now and then. Diet, regular massage and yoga therapy help to prevent headaches. When you are fatigued and have been stressed you should have a deep-tissue massage of the neck and shoulders to avoid severe headaches.

MIGRAINE

Migraine is a disease in which headache is one of the main symptoms. Not all headaches are migraine. The word migraine originated from two words, *hemi* – 'half' and *grania* – 'skull' or 'head'. Therefore one of its characteristic features is a half-sided headache. Typically, a migraine headache is characterised by the following symptoms: one-sided headache, nausea, photophobia (sensitivity to light), sensitivity to sound, light-headedness, aura or premonition of an attack (flashing lights, anxiety), vomiting, vertigo, fatigue after an attack, dizziness, palpitation or pulsating headache, hyperventilation (rapid breathing), scalp tenderness, fainting (occasional) and, occasionally, a confused state of mind.

Migraine, like chronic fatigue syndrome, is a collection of symptoms. Whereas headache is the lead symptom in one, fatigue is the predominant symptom in the other. There are other symptoms that go along with them.

Trigger factors

The actual cause of migraine is not known. It seems that many factors can trigger an attack, either individually or in combination. Some of these factors are:

- **hormonal changes** Women get migraine around the time of their periods.
- **vertebral artery compression** Neck stiffness causes compression of the vertebral arteries which trigger the headache and other symptoms by reducing the flow of blood to the brain stem. The brain stem has centres that control palpitation, hyperventilation, nausea, dizziness and so on.
- **stress** This may manifest itself by tensing up the neck muscles which in turn squeeze the vertebral artery on the vulnerable side and restrict circulation of brain fluid (CSF).

Coffee, cheese, milk, sugar, gluten, the smell of wet paint, shellfish or MSG can trigger a migraine attack in some people. These people must be sensitive to these substances to such a degree that as soon as they appear in the body, the reaction is there, because the body's tolerance limit has been crossed. Sometimes, however, it is not the intake of these substances that triggers the attack, but their withdrawal. People who are 'used to' or addicted to coffee, sleeping pills, alcohol or cigarettes suffer a tremendous headache, palpitation, nausea and so on when they suddenly stop using them. This is not a typical migraine attack but all the symptoms resemble it. The body doesn't like the change as it has adapted to the substances. I know a person who has a withdrawal-type migraine attack on the first couple of days of his holiday, when he switches off completely from all mental activities. Thus, although the timing of migraine attack is predictable, the actual cause or factors that trigger it is unknown.

Besides these factors there are other unknown causes. Since migraine attacks last for more than a day it seems that the cause has a prolonged effect on the body. It is as if a substance enters the body and the body takes two to three days to eliminate it from the blood. On the other hand, migraine is another example where the sanogenetic powers control the ailment even if no medicines are taken. If you have a migraine attack, you could sit in a dark room with a headband and wait for it to go away in two to three days. Vomiting dehydrates the body so you would need to drink enough water to compensate for that. In the days before powerful drugs were invented, this is how people treated themselves. In fact, when drugs are taken they only dull the headache, they do not cure it. Beta-blockers that slow the heart rate reduce the intensity of the headache.

Cluster migraines

In the case of cluster migraine, the causes seem even more intriguing. For a few months or weeks every year or every other year, the person will get a severe headache every day at a fixed time, several times a day. It is as if a time has been fixed in the body and the attacks come at a predetermined moment. Like sleep, body temperature (high at 4 p.m. and lower at 4 a.m.), menstrual periods, and physical or psychological peaks, migraine follows a certain biorhythm. Cluster migraine is a perfect example of this biorhythm, which in my opinion is an extension of all natural phenomena (day, month, year, seasons, climate and so on all follow a certain natural rhythm).

Cyclical patterns

We do see diseases occurring in certain rhythms. For example there is a flu season, a hay fever season, a stomach disorder season (summer), and a season for mental disease (spring, winter). It seems cluster migraine is seasonal since most people seem to get these headaches in spring and early summer for a period of about eight to twelve weeks. Some phenomena are taking place during this period which have a continuous ill effect on our health (see pages 150–151). The sanogenetic powers are too run down at this time of year to cope with the pathogenetic agents. The pollens being released into the air, the invading bacteria, viruses and fungal spores rising from the soil in response to the warmth of the sun thawing the snow, the positioning of the sun and other planets in relation to the earth – all these factors must be playing some role in our sensitive body system. While it deals with these on a routine basis, in springtime the sheer magnitude of the invading agents coupled with the general weakness of the sanogenetic powers tips the balance of the body.

If, logically speaking, what I argue is true, then the monthly or bimonthly migraine that most sufferers get must be the result of the effect of some external or environmental factor on the susceptible body. We all know there is a biorhythm in our body – there are moments when our physical and mental stamina is high and there are periods during the month when everything hits rock bottom. It is nature's way and cycles are essential proofs of that rule. You cannot be high all the time or else the body would never be able to cope and would get exhausted.

Whether it is a single episode of migraine or a cluster migraine, the rhythm of their occurrence points to something cyclical in nature. I have treated a famous French chef who used to get a migraine attack every Saturday at 11 p.m. It occured like clockwork, and he would spend the night in agony and the whole of Sunday in bed. I managed to break the chain and he began to get less intense attacks. Then he missed a few Saturdays and eventually they stopped altogether. The wife of a famous songwriter from Hollywood used to get her migraine at 6:30 p.m. every day. It took a few weeks to break this pattern and it is obvious that some internal and external factors played a role in triggering the attacks. I've tried very hard to find the common denominator to establish the cause of these attacks but have not so far succeeded. The human body is very complicated and that is why we have a tendency to put the cause down to stress or psychological problems. Some would argue that because patients expect a headache to start at a certain time they get it.

Preventing migraine attacks

Since the timing of a migraine attack can often be predicted, I plan my treatment so that people take precautions two to three days before the presumed date of attack. A preventive plan carried out over six to twelve months helps to break the pattern of migraine attacks. The attacks become less severe at first and then less frequent.

Regimen Therapy plays an important role a few days before the attack. To persuade people to practise prevention, however, is a very difficult task because the majority of those brought up in the culture of conventional medicine do not practise routine preventive measures. The attitude is 'we will see when it happens' and sometimes that is too late. People in general secure their future with health insurance, a pension fund, life insurance and so on, to make sure that in difficult times their financial status will be safeguarded. Yet when it comes to taking preventive measures to secure their health, they become indifferent. I think people should pay more attention to preventive measures for their own sake.

Diet

Approximately three days before the anticipated date of attack:

- do a fruit and vegetables fast for one day. It is best not to do a complete water fast, as this may trigger the attack by releasing the toxins in the body. Fasting very often causes headaches. Eat non-citrus fruits and raw vegetable salads (lettuce, cucumber, carrots, watercress, sprouts, etc.).

- on the remaining two days avoid coffee, sugar, cheese, milk, yeast products, shellfish, citrus fruits, all canned or preserved products, fried food, spicy food, nuts, MSG (e.g. in Chinese food) and alcohol.

Particular emphasis should be placed on avoiding acid foods (citrus fruits, vinegar, spicy foods, etc.). During a migraine attack there is nausea and vomiting, and excess acid in the stomach may increase this tendency. The body vomits to throw out fluids so the blood volume will decrease. This makes it possible for the fluid pressure in the brain to reduce, which eases the headache. So after vomiting the patient does get some relief.

Massage

At least once in the three-day period you must have a deep-tissue massage of the neck and shoulders. This will improve the flow of blood to the head. In any case, the neck stiffens up before a migraine attack and massage can help that situation tremendously.

Exercises

For three days it is advisable to spend 10–15 minutes each morning doing the general yoga exercises detailed on pages 64–73, followed by Shavasana (S4) or relaxation. Besides yoga, you should walk in the fresh air and swim if there is an opportunity.

Other measures

- Go to bed early – avoid late nights.
- Eat early (by 8 p.m. at the latest).
- Eat slowly.
- Avoid confrontational situations. As far as possible, avoid stressful situations.

Specific treatment

- **Acupuncture**
- **Homoeopathy** after consulting the specialist
- **Herbal remedies:** Valeriana drops, ten drops twice a day for three days
- **Head massage with Ayurvedic oils**
- **Osteopathic or chiropractic adjustments** or cranial osteopathy

For **cluster migraine**, precautions should be taken at least one month before the expected date of the attacks. The Regimen Therapy outlined above should be adhered to very strictly. It is best to do a total water fast one day per week for four to six weeks prior to the attacks.

Cluster migraine is a serious condition and therefore it is better to take preventive measures well in advance than wait for the headaches to start. Once they begin they are fairly difficult to control with self-help techniques.

Treatment

Migraine is one of the severest form of pain human beings suffer. When the attacks come, a person is completely out of action. All efforts should be made to control it immediately. Since it is an acute condition some immediate measures will have to be taken.

Diet

Eat very simply during migraine attacks. Vegetable soup, porridge with water, semi-boiled eggs, puréed vegetables, mashed potatoes, grilled fish, bananas, apples, pears and spinach are best eaten. Avoid everything else. The stomach is often churned up from vomiting and therefore needs easily digested foods.

Sip plenty of water between meals so that the nausea does not cause vomiting. Drink camomile and peppermint tea.

Other treatment

- Put a cold pack on your forehead.
- Put a hot-water bottle, wrapped in a towel, under your neck.
- Rest in bed as much as possible.
- Keep the windows open to allow fresh air in.

Massage

1

Gently massage the neck and shoulders. During a migraine attack this area will be extremely stiff. Ask somebody to massage it for five to ten minutes every two hours or so if the headache continues.

2

Ask somebody to put a towel under your neck while you are on your back. Ask him or her to gently grip your neck just below the back of your head and apply traction by pulling gently. Those with 'unstable' necks as a result of a previous trauma should always take care when using traction.

Relaxation

Practise Shavasana (S4) with full breathing exercises (rhythmic and slow), particularly B6 (see pages 64–73). This might help the nervous system to relax.

If all these treatments fail to relieve the pain within two hours, resort to conventional medicine.

Conventional medicine

New types of drug are very efficient in controlling migraine. Although they are expensive, they work quite quickly. Most of them make the blood less viscous or thick so that it can flow through the arteries to reach the brain membrane. The spasm of the arteries during an attack makes it very difficult for the blood to flow through them.

Oxygen is often used to relieve severe headache. Sometimes ozone therapy, which improves the oxygenation of brain tissue, helps to control the headache.

In the case of cluster migraine, Regimen Therapy and specialised treatments should be used alongside conventional medical treatment. A combination of osteopathy or chiropractic, acupuncture and massage of the neck and shoulders should reduce the intensity of the headaches as well as making them less frequent.

Prognosis

Migraine is a debilitating disease. It destroys the confidence of the sufferer. It is so unbearable that people are driven to the limit of their tolerance. Thanks to the new conventional drugs, these headaches are controllable. The drugs have side-effects, no doubt, but in times of acute crisis they are very useful. You must realise, however, that conventional drugs can do no more than control the headaches when they come – there is no cure for the disease, (except that when the menstrual periods stop in women, the headaches also stop in many cases).

The best hope is Regimen Therapy which, combined with acupuncture, osteopathy or homoeopathy, has shown good results, with the migraine attacks becoming less frequent. Remember that constant running down of the physis will lower the defences, allowing long-term pathogenic invasion, so any measure to reduce the onslaught of the disease is worthwhile.

Chapter 17

PSYCHOLOGICAL PROBLEMS
Stress

As I explained in Chapter 3, the relationship between mind and body is neglected in teaching medicine and therefore many psychological factors of disease are still today not taken significantly into account. One of these factors is stress.

'Stress' is one of the most common words used in today's urban society. Different people have tried to describe it and yet have not come to a definite answer. We all know what stress is but we cannot explain it in words that will cover all the aspects of it. In a way health is a similar condition in that it has no clear definition.

Different people experience stress differently so it is not measurable. Everything depends on one's tolerance threshold which is determined by the constitution and well-being. Medicine has tried to describe stress in general terms using some of the symptoms, as it has done with chronic fatigue syndrome, irritable bowel syndrome and so on. Therefore stress is really a syndrome which is multifactorial and the symptoms may or may not be related to each other.

Symptoms of stress

- **Sleep disturbances** Inability to fall asleep or waking up several times at night, especially around 3 or 4 a.m.
- **Irritability or depression** These symptoms depend on an individual's reaction.
- **Lack of concentration**
- **Short-term memory loss** What happened 15–20 minutes ago is not recalled. Long-term memory is good.
- **Hypervigilance** Always worrying about what other people are saying about you can be a symptom of stress.
- **Feeling detached or estranged** from others.
- **No hope** for the future.
- **Aches and pains**
- **Headaches, dizziness, tinnitus**
- **Loss of libido**
- **Increased startle response** (get startled very easily)
- **Loss of appetite** and other digestive problems (bloating, loose stools, constipation, etc.)
- **Mood fluctuations** (erratic behaviour)
- **Irregular periods in women**
- **Disturbing dreams** about death, financial misfortune, etc.
- **Fear** (as an emotional symptom which results from stress)
- **Palpitation and hyperventilation**
- **Panic attacks**
- **Tingling in the limbs**
- **Backache**

These physical and emotional symptoms cover most of the systems of the body – emotional, circulatory, respiratory, digestive, hormonal, musculo-skeletal and immunological. Therefore it is a multi-systemic disorder, affecting the mind and the body.

What is stress?

Stress became known through the work of the Canadian scientist Sele, who hypothesised that an external stimulus which acts as a threat or concern for the body causes the release of norephedrine (popularly known as adrenalin) from the two pea-sized glands located above the kidneys (adrenal glands). When this hormone is released into the bloodstream the sympathetic response of 'fight or flight' comes into play. The hormone is transported within seconds to every part of the body via the circulatory system. That is why the response is overwhelming and all parts of the body react simultaneously.

When a fox sees a dog both animals go through similar biochemical and hormonal changes but varying 'emotional' states. The dog is in a 'fight' state of mind, whereas the fox is in the 'flight' (fear) state. Yet their internal systems go through identical changes. The situation (stress) releases adrenalin which causes the following reactions in the body: increased heart rate (palpitation), breathing rate (hyperventilation) and metabolic rate (consumption of oxygen, burning of fat), and muscle tension. At this time both animals become 'automated' and do not focus on anything other than the situation they are in. This is an acute reaction and as soon as the situation improves (the animals lose sight of each other) the heightened responses return to the normal level one by one. The effects of stress are cured.

If this situation is repeated every day and is almost continuous, then the body gets conditioned and responds even when there is no obvious threat. Like the dogs in Pavlov's experiment that responded to noise and flickering lights by secreting stomach acid even though there wasn't any food associated with the stimuli, stress reactions become automatic. Instead of responding to the stressful situation only when it occurs, the body gets 'used to' the situation and produces the adrenalin anyway in expectation. That is what happens with continuous stress.

Unfortunately what happens as a physiological response in an acute stress situation becomes a permanent pathological condition. The constant release of stress hormones into the blood causes an increase in the pulse rate, and breathing rate, muscular tension and anxiety almost permanently. It is as if the body is in a stressful situation all the time. So even when the body tries to rest it cannot – the sleep is disturbed, the blood pressure is raised, the panic attacks come in the middle of the night, waking the person up. Unless he or she really tries to switch off and takes precautionary measures to combat this state, a condition develops which is highly dangerous to health.

What causes stress?

Conflict is at the root of most stress. A lot of stress is caused by dilemmas, having to decide between two conflicting aims: it's the most stressful thing a human being can face, like the hungry donkey between two haystacks. The other human menace is deadlines. The nervous system follows a certain rhythm and pattern. When you hurry it up you become stressed because the mind has its own cyclical pattern. You may be able to complete the work in a certain period but the moment you create a deadline you create stress. Deadlines and dilemmas are the two major causes of stress. They are an outside influence on the brain. Another serious form of stress comes from human relationships. Conflicts, clashes, quarrels, overcrowding, antisocial behaviour, people who tell you you are wrong (even when you are) and, especially, moving home and bereavement, all increase stress. Furthermore, nearly all stress derived from these situations is unavoidable.

On top of these are the avoidable sources of stress: builders hammering upstairs, noisy neighbours, people who turn up the volume on music you don't like, discomfort from driving over rough ground, flashing lights, having to take pills in a complicated programme. All these invasions of our senses can be highly stressful, although they are theoretically avoidable by shutting ourselves up in a dark, silent room.

On the other hand, we need some stress to generate the minimum or normal secretion of adrenalin, so necessary to keep us going, to unlock our storehouse of energy. Without stress there would be no adaptation, no response to any external or internal threat. In fact, life would be impossible. When you get up in the morning you would not be able to gear up for the day if your stress hormones weren't being actively secreted from the early hours of the morning (around 4 a.m.). Surgically removing the adrenal glands to eliminate stress hormones would be disastrous, as these are vital controllers of life processes. In acute medical conditions, like shock, severe allergic reaction, advanced autoimmune disease, cardiac arrest or respiratory failure, cortisone (or steroids) is injected. This is a form of stress hormone used for emergency medicine. Adrenalin is injected directly into the heart to 'kick-start' it when it stops beating and other resuscitation methods have failed. Thus stress hormones and in fact stress itself are vital to the body. In the end it all boils down to the same old thing – moderation and variety in all things, not just in our diet, but in stress factors as well.

The effects of stress on the body

There are scores of diseases which are linked to stress. These diseases include: psychological diseases, high blood pressure, psoriasis, cancer, certain forms of eczema, neurodermatitis, autoimmune diseases (rheumatoid arthritis, lupus, ulcerative colitis), weak immune system (Epstein Barr virus and postviral fatigue or ME, tuberculosis), and increased sensitivity to allergens (allergies). There are scores of other diseases which are indirectly linked to stress (such as complications arising from hypertension, addictions to alcohol or drugs, and eating disorders).

The links between stress and these diseases are not always clear, though I have my own hypothesis on the matter. The effects of stress on the body are shown in two ways, via primary pathways and secondary pathways.

The primary pathway is manifested by the effect of stress hormones on nerve receptors of the various organs, exhibited by high blood pressure, muscle tension, neurodermatitis, stomach ulcers, psoriasis, certain forms of eczema, irritable bowel syndrome (diarrhoea, constipation), backache and so on.

The secondary pathway of stress is manifested in the following way:

Stress / muscular tension / tightness of the neck muscles / decreased blood flow through vertebral arteries to the base of the brain and brain stem / malfunctioning of the nerve centres of the brain stem and base of brain (together known as the subconscious brain).

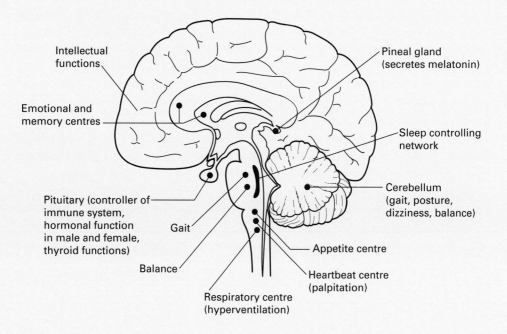

Intellectual functions

Emotional and memory centres

Pineal gland (secretes melatonin)

Sleep controlling network

Cerebellum (gait, posture, dizziness, balance)

Pituitary (controller of immune system, hormonal function in male and female, thyroid functions)

Gait

Balance

Appetite centre

Heartbeat centre (palpitation)

Respiratory centre (hyperventilation)

Results of malfunction at brain stem

- Panic attacks (palpitation and hyperventilation)
- Headaches
- Tinnitus
- Dizziness
- Craving for food
- Bell's palsy
- Sleep disturbances
- Nausea, vomiting (in acute stress)

Results of malfunction at base of brain

- Emotional problems (anxiety, lack of concentration, poor memory, fear, hypervigilance, hypersensitivity, irritability, mood swings)
- Malfunction of hypothalamus and pituitary gland, irregular periods, weak immune system, loss of libido
- Lack of motivation
- Poor melatonin secretion, causing restlessness at night

Thus the secondary or indirect effect of stress also leads to the manifestation of many diseases.

Stress signals from sensory nerves (vision, hearing, smell, pain, discomfort, etc.) and intuitive receptors (telepathy, clairvoyance) are interpreted in the brain's analysing centres (frontal lobe), and then messages are sent to the base of the brain (hypothalamus and pituitary gland). Here control hormones (ACTH) are secreted into the blood and these reach the adrenal glands and stimulate the secretion of the various stress hormones. Thus the conscious brain receives the first signals on the stressful situation and passes the messages down.

These signals may not go through the conscious brain all the time. They may be recorded at the level of the subconscious and similar messages are sent for identical responses. The signals could be geopathic stress (from powerful electric cables running near the house, or the presence of electronic gadgets all around), environmental stress (high pollen count, extreme weather conditions, GM foods, pesticides, noise pollution, air pollution), or stress due to chronic diseases. These unseen or unrecorded stresses are the most difficult to deal with, as often they go unnoticed and the alarm is sounded only when stress is manifested in the form of disease.

Fatigue is a result of chronic stress. When the body is run down, there is a power failure and all the organs and systems function at low intensity. The digestion is sluggish, the elimination is poor, the muscles are listless, mind capacity is reduced and the immune system is weak. When all these conditions occur over a long period, the adrenal glands become completely exhausted. You head either for a 'nervous breakdown' or total exhaustion. Once this happens only an active and well-planned treatment can revitalise the body and mind once again.

Stress may not always cause physical symptoms. Sometimes it remains within the boundaries of the conscious brain and does not extend to the lower (subconscious) part of the brain. In psychiatry we find thousands of patients with heavy-duty mental problems (paranoia, obsession, thought persecution, fear of death, violent manic attacks, depression, etc.) but they have hardly any physical problems. It is as if Mother Nature has spared them from physical suffering as they are in deep mental agony.

In cases of anorexia and bulimia, patients inflict upon themselves severe nutritional deficiencies. These cause many physical problems – osteoporosis, poor immune system, low blood pressure, loss of hormonal function (loss of menstruation), yet the 'mental energy' in anorexics is so great that despite their poor nutritional status, they are able to take vigorous exercise without signs of fatigue or exhaustion. They have severe weight loss and their bones are so brittle as a result of calcium deficiency that exercise causes fractures. Yet they do not feel the pain from these obvious problems of the bones and joints. Their mind is in a different sphere. Stress immunises them against physical pain and discomfort.

The important thing about stress is that if the body is able to return its abnormal functions to normal level, then stress does not cause any lasting health problems.

Stress management

This is perhaps one of the few medical conditions that requires management rather than treatment. We need a certain amount of stress to survive but we do not want it to have permanent or severe effects on our health. In other words, stress has to be policed so that it does not go out of control and cause disruption.

In order to manage stress two golden rules have to be followed:

1   **Improve the threshold of tolerance of stress**
2   **Carry out damage control of the effects of stress**

Both these goals can comfortably be achieved by carrying out **Regimen Therapy** fairly strictly. They say 'the body is the temple of the mind'. A nice clean body maintained to meet the energy demands put upon it can nurture a healthy mind. 'Mind over matter is matter undermined' and by looking after the physical self you can keep the mind clear and stress-free. Some American workaholics use the principle 'Work hard and work out hard', meaning that by taking regular exercise you can work very hard and deal with a lot of stress.

Diet

Avoid coffee, excess salt, yeast products, excess alcohol (small amounts of diluted spirits can relax), canned products, cheese, mushrooms, excess citrus juices, MSG as in Chinese food, fried food and very spicy food.

Drink more carrot and apple juice, camomile tea and ginger tea. You should also drink plenty of water, as stress dehydrates the body.

Lifestyle changes

- Avoid eating fast. Always sit down to eat.
- Avoid late nights and get plenty of sleep. Eat dinner early.
- Do not watch disturbing films before going to bed.
- Have frequent breaks when working with computers for long hours, as they tighten the neck and create great stress.
- Use holidays and weekends to replenish energy.

Massage

This is an excellent way to release physical and emotional stress. The deep-tissue massage with more emphasis on the neck and shoulders can help to alleviate physical and emotional signs of stress. Sometimes a good therapeutic massage can release spasms in muscles, improve circulation of blood to the brain and therefore invigorate it, remove aches and pains in the muscles and the back, and induce relaxation. If you are in a stressful situation, you should have a deep-tissue massage therapy once or twice a month.

Exercises

Yoga is excellent for stress because of its emphasis on breathing and relaxation, so the general exercises and Shavasana (S4), detailed on pages 64–73 are recommended. Breathing correctly eliminates signs of stress. Symptoms like palpitation and hyperventilation, which appear so frequently in stress, are cured very quickly with controlled breathing. Besides yoga, aerobic exercises, jogging and Pilates are good for stress. Walking is an excellent form of exercise for stress management. This should be done in a place where there is plenty of fresh air. This is why I conduct my Stress Management Programme in the Himalayas. I have been doing this for almost 12 years with groups of my patients. I hardly need add that they have yoga and massage every day. Also walking in remote areas and coming into contact with different tribal culture and lifestyle helps to detach yourself from the everyday life that you find stressful.

Medicines

1 **Homoeopathy**
2 **Acupuncture**
3 **Nutritional medicine** – B-complex, magnesium (relaxes the body), occasional infusions of vitamins and minerals
4 **Herbal medicines:**
   - Ginseng (one capsule per day)
   - Ayurvedic mixture – Shankh Puspi, Jatamansi, Ashwagandha in equal proportion, either in tablet form or in powder form in infusions (teabags)

Meditation

This is often covered by Shavasana of the yoga programme (see page 68). If you are very stressed, you should do this exercise separately in the evening.

Psychological therapies

1 **Neurolinguistic Programming** (NLP) This is a psychiatric treatment which uses words to help to re-programme the thought process and alleviate stress
2 **Psychoanalysis and psychotherapy**
3 **Group therapy**

Conventional medicines

Conventional medicine should be used in extreme cases. The medicines of choice are:

- Mild antidepressants
- Sleeping tablets
- Beta-blockers (to slow down the heart)
- Mild anti-anxiety medicine

Prognosis

Stress can be managed, and if you are very susceptible to it, you should follow a certain lifestyle or Regimen Therapy all the time. Stress causes many critical diseases and therefore it has to be taken very seriously and controlled.

Chapter 18

THE HORMONAL/REPRODUCTIVE SYSTEM
Infertility and menstrual problems

Problems affecting the hormonal system can be far reaching and many of the body's other systems can suffer. If the problem is confined to the reproductive system, however, the body might otherwise function normally. An example of such a relatively confined disorder is infertility, a distressing complaint to both partners, but nevertheless not directly affecting their general health.

INFERTILITY

Male and female infertility is on the rise in urban society, especially in the West. At a time when the population is booming in some parts of the world, there are people who cannot conceive at all. Some cry for babies whereas others wish they were not so fertile. Some reports seem to indicate that there is a decrease in male sperm counts and an increasing number of menstrual problems in women. With the new technology available, low sperm count is not an insurrmountable difficulty because sperm can be concentrated and used to fertilise eggs. The motility (ability to swim fast) of the sperm is a more significant problem.

Female infertility

Controlling infertility in women with technology is difficult since there are various factors involved. The drugs used to stimulate ovulation cause many disturbing side-effects (physical and psychological) and are potentially harmful to the body, and yet women put themselves through such treatment in the hope that the miracle might happen. It seems that only 10 out of every 100 who try this uncomfortable method manage to conceive. Some go to great lengths, spending every penny and selling homes to be able to afford the treatment. Some women feel that they are incomplete if they do not have a child. The social stigma attached to infertility can be immense. More complications start if family members demand a grandchild, in particular a son to continue the family name. This pressure can be very disturbing for a woman, especially if her partner is not very understanding.

Causes of infertility

1

Lack of ovulation and maturation of the egg cell This results from ovarian and hormonal problems.

2

Blocked fallopian tubes Blockage of the tubes that carry the egg to the uterus can result from infection or can be congenital.

3

Poor thickening of the lining of the uterus If the lining is thin then the fertilised egg is unable to implant in the uterus. The thickness of the lining is mainly determined by the hormones oestrogen and progesterone. If their concentration in the blood is low then there are complications.

4

Poor general health If Nature feels that a woman is unfit to bear a child because of poor general health (anorexia or anaemia, for example) then she will not allow her to conceive because of the high risk to mother and foetus.

5

Small uterus

Indirect causes

1

Stress This is foremost amongst the general indirect causes of infertility. Firstly, stress causes tightness in the neck muscles, affecting blood flow through the vertebral arteries to the pituitary gland. When the pituitary gland malfunctions, the hormones that stimulate ovulation (FSH) are not secreted in sufficient quantity. Ovulation may be delayed as a result, making the menstrual cycle longer or erratic. Secondly, stress can cause contraction of the fallopian tubes or the uterine muscles. In the first case the egg may not be able to reach the sperm cells and in the second case implantation of the fertilised egg may not be able to take place.

Stress can cause involuntary spasms. The 'nervous gut' syndrome, for example, is nothing but spasms of the intestines due to stress. High blood pressure is caused by constriction of blood vessels. Therefore it is very likely that the uterine muscles and the fallopian tubes can go into spasm because of stress. Since the blood flow to the inner lining of the uterus (endometrium) goes through layers of muscle, spasm there cuts off this vital supply. Reduced blood supply to the endometrium can lead to its malnourishment and make it difficult for the fertilised egg (if there is any) to settle in. This leads to a failed pregnancy.

2

Infection, presence of fibroids in the uterus, endometriosis (when the inner lining of the uterus spreads into other tissue) are some of the other factors that interfere with the implanting of the fertilised egg.

3

Neck problems In response to an article published in the *Daily Mail* on my fertility treatment, some 70 women came to see me. Over 50 of them operated computers and complained of neck tension. Computers cause stress which in turn reduces cerebral circulation causing fatigue, panic attacks, pituitary malfunction and subsequent hormonal malfunction.

4

Easy bruising Women who bruise easily may have difficulty in retaining the fertilised egg on the matured endometrium. Mild liver function caused by prolonged use of contraceptive pills, alcohol or drug abuse etc. may cause easy bruising.

5

Excessive exercise and physical training Sportswomen and exercise instructors frequently have difficulty conceiving. This is probably due to the muscle-building hormones which have traits of male hormones and act like the contraceptive pill.

Treatment of female infertility

Infertility treatment should be carried out in two ways:

1   **General or Regimen Therapy**
2   **Specific treatment of the causes of infertility**

Regimen Therapy plays an important role in the treatment of infertility. It not only regulates the natural menstrual cycle but also manages stress as well. These are the two most important factors in the infertility treatment.

Diet

Avoid citrus fruits, garlic in excess, spicy food, canned products, yeast products, coffee, alcohol, sugar, fried food and fizzy drinks. Citrus juices, spicy food and garlic may change the pH level of the vaginal area. The medium may become too acidic in which case it will act like a spermicide. Fizzy water, yeast products and canned foodstuffs may produce excess abdominal gas and thus disturb the circulation in the pelvic area.

When trying to tackle a problem of infertility, make sure your diet includes the following:

- **Pomegranate** This was traditionally recommended for infertility by certain herbalists in India. If you were to look at a pomegranate seed under a magnifying glass you would see that it has the shape of a uterus with a small spherical bulb in the centre, representing the foetus. Thus the pomegranate seed looks like the uterus of a pregnant woman. Perhaps nature gave some hint through this incredible shape and structure that the fruit is good for women who are either pregnant or trying to become pregnant.

  What active ingredients are present in pomegranate that help pregnancy is not specifically known, but we do know that this fruit has a high level of cobalt. That is why the colour of pomegranate fruit is purple – cobalt red. Cobalt is an essential element of haemoglobin in blood (present as cobalamine) and it is this part that absorbs and transports oxygen. Cobalt is therefore the essential raw material for synthesis of blood, and an important element for pregnant women.

Throughout pregnancy women take iron and folic acid to keep the blood synthesis going but they forget an essential microelement like cobalt in food.

Pomegranate also has a high iron content. This also helps blood synthesis, a process that is vital for women of reproductive age.

- **Apples, carrots and other fruit** for vitamins and minerals
- **High-protein diet** This is important as protein is essential for the reproductive function of a woman. Synthesis of blood and hormones, development of egg cells in the ovaries and growth of the inner lining of the womb involve proteins and they cannot be wholly replaced by other foodstuffs. Animal proteins (fish, chicken, eggs) are preferable to vegetable proteins, especially as oestrogen is synthesised from a cholesterol-based product found only in animal fat protein. In fact, cellulite deposits in women help to supplement the level of estrogen in the blood when it is low. Therefore, fat and estrogen production are strongly linked.

Massage

Massage of the neck and spine is very essential in infertility treatment. Not only does this create a 'feelgood' factor, it actually helps to reduce stress. Massage of the neck and shoulder area helps to reinstate blood flow to the brain stem and the pituitary gland. This in turn helps to improve the functioning of hormones such as FSH. Specific massage of the abdominal area has a therapeutic effect on the uterus and tubes by improving blood flow.

Yoga exercises

The general yoga exercises on pages 64–73 are useful, but full Cobra (P1), Turtle (M2), Semi bridge (S3), Child Pose (S1), Abdominal Massage (E2), Breathing while squatting (M1), are particularly beneficial. Shavasana (S4) after the other exercises is especially effective in relieving stress.

Specific treatments

1 **Homoeopathy and acupuncture** Both these therapies could be useful in reducing stress.
2 **Herbal remedies**
   Mix together 1 teaspoon of Shatavari powder, 1/2 teaspoon of Kolonji oil, 7–8 saffron leaves and 1 teaspoon of honey. Take with warm milk after breakfast.
   - **Mexican yam capsules** Take 1 capsule per day from the fourteenth day of the cycle until your period starts. This will help to thicken the lining of the uterus.

Male infertility

About one third of infertility problems originate from the male. Low sperm count, poor motility (mobility) and fewer living sperms account for the main problems related to male infertility. This has nothing to do with loss of sexual functions as in impotence.

Treatment of male infertility

To improve sperm count, stress management through **Regimen Therapy** is essential. Follow the same plan as for female infertility. In addition:

- **Egg flip** Take a raw farm egg (organic) and break into a glass of hot creamy milk. Stir up to make an egg flip. Add salt and pepper to taste. Drink at breakfast. This increases sperm production. Always make sure the egg comes from a good source or is organic, to avoid salmonella poisoning.

- **Herbal remedies** Mix a pinch of asafoetida, 1 teaspoonful of Ashwagandha (Indian ginseng), a match-head sized piece of Shilajit (minerals from the Himalayas, rich in zinc and magnesium) and 1/2 teaspoonful of powdered ginger. Add a little honey and take with milk once a day after a meal.

General recommendations

1

Stop worrying about not conceiving. The more you worry the more stressed you get. As experience has shown, women who have tried to conceive for years do so only when they cease to try. Often, when a couple adopt a child the woman then becomes pregnant.

2

Do not do strenuous work like lifting and carrying and avoid high-impact exercises such as weightlifting and jogging. Yoga is subtle and relaxing.

3

Around ovulation time, the twelfth to fifteenth day, avoid excitement of all types. Do relaxation breathing (B6) twice a day for 10–15 minutes and Shavasana (S4). Drink plenty of water, and eat lots of protein, fresh fruit and vegetables. An additional boost of vitamins and minerals during this phase is good.

4

Have intercourse in the early hours of the morning after a good night's sleep. Lie in bed for at least an hour after intercourse. Go to bed early on the previous night. Nowadays, there are simple tests available to tell you when you ovulate. Intercourse on the day of ovulation or the following day is very good. In fact, refrain from sexual contact for a week before the expected ovulation day so as to 'mature' the sperms.

5

Try to conceive before your fortieth birthday. The chances of success are always better.

MENSTRUAL PROBLEMS

Most women suffer some kind of menstrual problem at some stage in their lives. Menstruation is a natural function and it should occur every month without any problem. If problems do occur, it is an indication of some abnormal condition within the body.

Menstrual cycles are like the lunar calendar, approximately 28 days (4 weeks) long. The cycle is counted from the day the period starts (day one). Normally the bleeding lasts from three to five days. Soon afterwards, with the help of oestrogen secreted from the ovaries, the lining of the uterus begins to thicken and reaches its maximum thickness on approximately the fourteenth day. Around this time, a mature egg cell is produced from the ovary. This is called ovulation. At this time the body temperature goes up, sweat production and vaginal discharge increase and a woman may feel unusually anxious.

The egg is captured by the funnel of the fallopian tube, which directs it into the uterus. If fertilisation does not take place then this egg cell is useless.

The progesterone level increases initially to prepare the lining of the uterus to accept the fertilised egg. If fertilisation does not take place, the progesterone level suddenly drops. This withdrawal of progesterone causes the breaking down of the lining of the uterus and the cells, new blood vessels and blood are expelled in the form of menstruation.

The time during which a woman can conceive is approximately two days before ovulation and three to five days after ovulation. In a 28-day cycle, if ovulation takes place on the fourteenth day, then conception can take place between the twelfth and fourteenth day. Sperms live for four to five days. So if intercourse takes place any time between the twelfth and nineteenth day of the cycle, conception can take place. During all other times (before the twelfth day and after the nineteenth day) a woman is safe and free of risk of pregnancy. I must warn that there are individual variations. What I have said is taken on the basis that the woman has a 28-day cycle. It will be different for a woman with a 24-day or 32-day cycle. You must know when ovulation takes place in a particular month to be able to predict the safe (usually three days before ovulation and five days after ovulation) and unsafe periods in the cycle. For those who want a baby identifying when ovulation will take place is of paramount importance.

Menstrual periods start at around 11–13 years of age and stop at around 48–50 years. This is called the reproductive age. On average, women have periods for 36 years and to have a cycle of 26–28 days for all this time is not possible. After childbirth or surgical operations involving the lining of the uterus (D and C and abortion) the cycles can be altered. Stress, heavy physical work, anaemic conditions and malnutrition are also factors that can affect the menstrual cycle.

Menstrual problems

1

Excessive and prolonged bleeding Normally the menstrual period should last for three to four days with heavy bleeding lasting for the first couple of days. Sometimes the period lasts for ten days or so. This can happen because the lining is not regenerating quickly enough or because the clotting system is not working perfectly. Sometimes fibroids (fibrous knots or lumps in the uterine wall), low oestrogen level, infection in the uterus, the presence of an irritating contraceptive device (a coil for example) can cause such abnormal bleeding.

2

Bleeding between periods Something must be wrong if there is bleeding in between periods and it is advisable to see your doctor without delay. Erosions or ulcers in the neck of the uterus or infections can cause bleeding in midcycle. Since it is difficult to establish what is a normal period and what is not, it may seem that the periods are coming too soon. If abnormal bleeding starts on day 14 of the cycle, for example, it might be misinterpreted as an early period, since the bleeding is the main recognisable sign of periods.

3

Premenstrual syndrome (PMS) This is one of the worst complex of symptoms a woman can have. The symptoms may include: swollen and painful breasts, water retention, headaches, hot sweats, mood fluctuations, migraine headaches, nausea, chronic fatigue and depression.

When the womb is swollen and full of blood due to the thickened lining, there is pelvic congestion. The blood is rushed to the pelvis and this causes a reduced blood supply to the brain. Symptoms like fatigue, nausea, headaches and depression can result. It is rather like the situation when, after a heavy meal, the blood rushes to the intestines and similar symptoms are experienced.

The pelvic congestion causes sluggishness in the circulation of blood. This may cause water retention and bloating in the body and discomfort in the lower abdomen.

As soon as the periods start all these symptoms are relieved instantly. This clearly indicates that the pelvic congestion is the main contributory factor to the premenstrual symptoms. Treatments that improve circulation (like therapeutic yoga) help to relieve PMS.

4

Dysmenorrhoea (painful periods) Dysmenorrhoea is another uncomfortable symptom that precedes menstruation. Sometimes the abdominal cramp can be so severe that women pass out. There are various causes of this pain. One of the most common is the flexion or bending of the uterus, either forward or backward – normally the uterus stays upright. In certain women it is bent, mainly because of weakened ligaments that should bind and pull the uterus upright. When this happens there is a 'kink' in the uterine pathway near the bottom. Just before the period starts, the blood accumulates in the uterus without being able to ooze out of the opening at the bottom. The 'kink' or 'bend' prevents that from happening and so the uterine muscles begin to contract as if in labour to push the blood out. This contraction can go on for hours till at a certain stage, the blood is pushed out, relieving the uterine pressure instantly. The woman gets immediate relief as the contractions stop.

Sometimes infections in the uterus or a contraceptive device placed in it can trigger off mild contractions and can cause pain. These pains are not always linked to the periods.

5

Amenorrhoea (lack of periods) Sometimes teenage girls or adult women have no periods for months. Many are happy that they don't have to bother about hygiene and contraception whereas others are very concerned as they feel that a part of womanhood is missing. If a girl has never had periods then there is some defect in the reproductive system. Either the hormones are not in order or the uterus has some defects. It could be extremely small in size or the opening might be closed. These can be easily checked by investigation. This type of lack of periods is called **primary amenorrhoea**.

It is common for women to suffer from **secondary amenorrhoea,** which is when, after having regular cycles, the periods stop for six months or so. Again, women have mixed feelings about it. They have fully developed organs like breasts and the skin and voice are feminine, so they are not as worried as someone whose hormonal systems have not developed so well.

Stress is a common cause of this secondary amenorrhoea. Excessive stress causes secretion of stress hormones which by nature are like male hormones. These upset the natural equilibrium or balance between male and female hormones in the body. In my opinion this is what disrupts the periods.

Malnutrition, as in anorexia nervosa, causes chronic protein and mineral deficiency. Animal protein contains vitamin E which helps the periods, and more oestrogen is synthesised from certain fat and protein chains found in animal products. When anorexics shun animal products (eggs, fish, meat) totally, they create deficiencies that ultimately lead to reduced oestrogen production. The result is secondary amenorrhoea.

Problems affecting the ovaries like lack of ovulation, polycystic ovaries (multiple cysts on the ovary which replace the vital hormone-producing tissue and cause a decrease in oestrogen level) and infection or inflammation may cause lack of menstruation. It must be remembered that stress causes spasms of neck muscles which in turn reduce blood flow through the vertebral arteries in the neck. The decreased blood flow through these arteries may cause the pituitary gland to malfunction. The pituitary stimulates the ovaries to secrete oestrogen and therefore its malfunction disrupts the production of this hormone.

6

Leucorrhoea This is quite a common problem. A white or yellowish discharge flows freely out of the uterus and may produce a very strong 'rotting' smell. It is an uncomfortable condition and may require the use of sanitary protection. The most common cause is a bacterial or fungal infection (often causing thrush).

General treatment

In modern society having periods does not interfere with one's life, but in ancient times women took a lot of care during their periods. In fact in certain religious and cultural systems, there were rules that prevented women from going out during their periods, doing domestic work, visiting temples or mosques, eating heavy food and so on. Some restrictions were applied because menstruation was considered to be 'dirty'. In the Zoroastrian culture of ancient Persia, having sexual intercourse during menstruation was punishable by law. I advise the following during periods:

- avoid lifting heavy weights
- bath twice a day with lukewarm water (not very hot)
- refrain from sexual activities
- sleep early
- avoid late dinners.

Diet

- **Avoid** coffee, excess alcohol, excess salt, yeast products, sugars and sweets, fried food, spicy food, citrus juices, canned products and MSG.
- **Before periods:** eat vegetarian food and fish, fresh fruits, melon juice and nettle tea (to reduce water retention), camomile tea (for relaxation) and spinach soup. Eat light meals. Especially avoid fizzy water, rich and oily food, red meat, fried food and alcohol. Avoid smoking.
- **During periods:** drink a lot of water, soups (chicken, spinach), carrot juice, easily digested foods (mushy, slightly overcooked – mashed potatoes, minced meat, tofu), high protein diet (egg, fish, meat, soya products).
- **After periods:** eat more protein, spinach, non-citrus fruits, carrot juice, pomegranate and raw salad. Drink a lot of water, soups, ginger tea and ginseng tea. The idea is to build up the blood as soon as possible and tone up the blood pressure if it tends to be low.

Massage

A few days before your period starts, massages of the neck and shoulder area are beneficial. Ask your partner to massage you for five to ten minutes before you go to bed, especially when you go through premenstrual syndrome. An hour's treatment by a professional masseur is very beneficial a day or two before the expected date of menstruation. The massage eases up the tension in the neck and shoulders and improves the blood flow to the brain. It also has a calming effect on the nervous system.

Exercises

Therapeutic yoga exercises are very beneficial in treating various problems related to menstrual problems, in particular PMS. The following exercises are very important: Cobra (P1), Turtle (M2), Semi-Bridge (S3), Abdominal Massage (E2), Shavasana (S4). See pages 66–73 for these exercises.

Specific treatments

Premenstrual Syndrome (PMS)

- Homoeopathy
- Acupuncture (especially before menstruation)
- Vitamin and mineral infusions or oral vitamin B6, magnesium
- Ayurvedic remedies: 1 teaspoon of Shankh Pupsi mixed with 1 teaspoon of Shatavari powder, with water
- Hot tub baths with aromatic oils like lavender.

Amenorrhoea

- Homoeopathy
- Acupuncture
- Ayurvedic and other herbal combinations. Take the following mixture with warm milk or water, after breakfast daily: 1 teaspoon of Shatavari, 1/2 teaspoon of kolongi oil, 7–8 saffron leaves, 1 teaspoon of honey, 1 tablespoon of protein powder (if vegetarian). To complement this medicine take two capsules of aloe vera daily.

In addition to the above combination which in general improves oestrogenic functions, take one or two capsules of Mexican yam between the fifteenth and thirtieth of each calendar month. Mexican yam is a mimic for progesterone, acting similarly in the body. Shatavari and kolonji also have oestrogenic properties. They mimic the action of oestrogen but have no recorded side-effects.

Dysmenorrhoea

- Homoeopathy
- Acupuncture
- Massage of the lower abdomen with sesame and camphor oils. Take a tablespoon of sesame oil and add a few drops of camphor oil and massage the lower abdomen in a clockwise fashion for a few minutes. Do this twice a day, starting one week before the period starts.
- If the pain starts always use a hot-water bottle (not an ice-pack) wrapped in a towel and placed on the lower abdomen.
- Do not use cold water to shower. Use warm baths. Remember that heat helps to relax the muscles of the uterus, which in principle should ease the tension.
- During the actual cramping acupuncture could be beneficial.
- The following Ayurvedic combination is recommended for three days before

menstruation: 1 teaspoon each of Ajwain (Phychotis Ajwain) and aniseed, with 10 gm of sliced raw ginger. Boil the above mixture for five minutes in about 250 ml of water and drink with or without honey in the morning. Repeat this concoction once again in the evening. This is an anti-spasmodic preparation. It relaxes the muscles of the womb.

A traditional Russian folk remedy for severe abdominal cramp before the onset of menstruation is: 'Drink 1/2 glass of vodka and sit in a hot tub with sea salt and mustard paste'. It is harsh treatment and I would not recommend it. I have mentioned it only to show how tension and spasm in the lower abdomen is traditionally recognised and relieved.

Leucorrhoea

- Homoeopathy
- Ayurvedic medicine – Supari Pak (betelnut paste) has the unusual property of contracting the uterine muscles. This results in the closing of the entrance to the uterus, thereby reducing the flow of the discharge.
- Conventional medicine – antibiotics or anti-fungal preparations.

Prognosis

Premenstrual syndrome, dysmenorrhoea, amenorrhoea and leucorrhoea are largely treatable. Treatment requires commitment on the part of the patient as the Regimen Therapy has to be strictly followed.

Chapter 19

THE DIGESTIVE SYSTEM
Acidity, Irritable bowel syndrome, Flatulence

The digestive system probably has the most direct influence of all the body's systems on your health. The moment you put something in your mouth there is an impact on health, positive or negative. The digestive system is the warehouse for the whole body, supplying nutrients to every other system. It is also their rubbish dump, being responsible for the disposal of most of the body's waste products. There is much that can go wrong and when it does it affects the whole body. It is probably true to say that the digestive system is the most abused system in the body. Things can go wrong in the warehouse, such as acidity, and in the dump, such as irritable bowel syndrome or flatulence.

ACIDITY

Causes

Heartburn is caused by regurgitation of excess acid from the stomach. When there is a lot of acid in the stomach, some of it comes up with burping into the food pipe and the mouth. This causes a tremendous burning sensation in the chest. Sometimes the acid may be accidentally sprinkled into the windpipe and the lungs causing burning and great discomfort in the entire chest area. The acid in the stomach is hydrochloric acid. Its excess production is caused by the following factors:

1

Diet Food must be the main cause of acid production since the purpose of the acid is to aid digestion. Certain foods aggravate this acid production. These are:
- fried and spicy food
- citrus fruits
- nuts and rough food (excessive movement of the stomach muscles is needed to churn these to a pulp)
- alcohol
- steaming hot tea, food and other drinks (these irritate the stomach lining).

2

Smoking or chewing tobacco Nicotine produces excess acid in the stomach.

3

Drugs Certain types of medicine such as aspirin, other painkillers and steroids produce inflammation of the stomach lining and therefore more acid is secreted.

4

Bacterial infection A type of bacteria known as helicobacter pylori thrives in the lining of the stomach, causing gastritis and ulcers. The resulting inflammation causes excess acid production.

5

Stress As proved by Pavlov in his classic experiments with dogs, stress produces excess acid secretion.

6

Eating fast When one eats fast, the food is dumped in the stomach without being properly chewed. This food mass has to be turned into a pulp before it is digested. To do this the stomach walls work extra hard and soften the food mass with acid secretion.

When I was a medical student some 22 years ago, people used to suffer from a condition called 'anhydric gastritis'. In this the level of acid secretion in the stomach was very low. Today such a condition is unheard of. Our eating habits have changed and therefore there is more acid production in the stomach than there used to be. Chillies and other spices were used in hot countries to stimulate appetite, which used to be low in the heat. Later these exotic spices were used to camouflage the smell of rotten meat and fish when refrigeration was not available. Today, when these spices are fried in excess oil to flavour food, they act as stimulators of gastric juices. One sweats, has excess saliva and frequently has heartburn. Also, high stress levels contribute to excess acid production.

Before the discovery of helicobacter pylori and the part it plays in acid production, drugs that suppressed acid production in the stomach were bestsellers. Antacids are still the largest selling drugs after painkillers. Therefore acidity and heartburn must be a significant problem for many people.

Treatment and prevention

All the causes mentioned above indicate that lifestyle changes can bring about great relief in controlling acidity and heartburn. If you eat the right type of food and eat it slowly, you will automatically be able to control this problem.

Diet

By eating the right type of food, and eating slowly, you can control the problem of excess acid. **Avoid** the following: citrus fruits, vinegar, fried and spicy food, canned products (because they contain excess vinegar), white wine, champagne, brandy, cider, excess tea or coffee, pineapples, excess tomatoes, fizzy canned drinks.

You should also avoid: painkillers, aspirin (unless coated), steroid tablets where possible, smoking, excess vitamin C (above 1 gram), excess zinc tablets (above 15 mg) and other supplements in large amounts.

General advice

- Eat slowly. Chew food well.
- Drink water 30–45 minutes after meals. Sip water during meals.
- Rest for 10–15 minutes after lunch and walk for 10 minutes after dinner.
- Avoid late dinners (especially near bedtime).
- Avoid fizzy water with main meals.

Medication

1 **Homoeopathy** for acidity
2 **Acupuncture** for acidity
3 **Ayurvedic herbal remedies:**
   - Shankh bhasm (This is a pure form of crystallized calcium carbonate, taken as a powder. It is made from seashells and is a powerful antacid.)
   - Avipattikar churna (herbal powder)
   - Peppermint oil
4 **Conventional medicine** This should be used when the acidity problem is high. There are blood tests that can show the presence of helicobacter in the gut. This should be treated with a course of antibiotics followed by a strict **Regimen Therapy** to boost the body's immune system.

Prognosis

Gastritis and hyperacidity can be easily treated. If chronic gastritis is not treated, the risk of stomach ulcers is great. These can turn into malignant tumours (stomach cancer).

IRRITABLE BOWEL SYNDROME

Irritable bowel syndrome (IBS) in my opinion is a vague name given to a range of symptoms that occur in the digestive system. Like ME (Myalgic Encephelomyalitis), chronic fatigue syndrome, stress, premenstrual syndrome and so on, it is a general condition consisting of related or unrelated symptoms.

Symptoms

IBS is characterised by the following symptoms:

1 Abdominal pain relieved by passage of stools
2 Flatulence

3 Frequent stools or constipation
4 Heartburn or indigestion
5 Burping and bloating shortly after a meal

Causes

Before diagnosing IBS physicians have to exclude a range of diseases and other conditions that may cause one or more of these symptoms. These are:

1 Parasites (giardiasis, amoebiasis)
2 Infection of the bowels
3 Ulcerative colitis (Crohn's disease)
4 Lactose or gluten intolerance
5 Thyrotoxicosis – hyperfunction of the thyroid gland (which causes diarrhoea)
6 Antibiotics, some blood pressure medicines
7 Psychological problems like depression and panic attacks (which causes nervous gut, diarrhoea)
8 Endometriosis
9 Colon cancer
10 Kidney failure (excess urea irritates the bowels)

If these diseases are not present and the cause of the symptoms is not known, IBS can be diagnosed. But because the cause is not known it is difficult to follow the principle of cause and effect in treating it. The only options left are (a) candidiasis (b) yeast-overgrowth in the gut (c) unknown causes. The candida or yeast overgrowth is identified with great difficulty and their role in IBS is heavily disputed by conventional medicine, even though avoiding yeast products improves the symptoms. There could be other causes such as deficiencies of vitamins and minerals (for example, vitamin B deficiency may cause the gut to be irritable), excessive supplement or drug intake (when they interact with each other), chemicals and preservatives in food, excess bile secretion (bile salts increase bowel movements), coffee or alcohol toxicity or diverticulitis (swelling of the colon with large storage areas).

When so many factors are involved, IBS is best treated as a multifactorial problem. The interesting fact about IBS is that both diarrhoea and constipation are considered as qualifying symptoms, even though both have diverse causes and are principally opposite to each other.

Most physicians consider IBS to be a psychological problem as they cannot identify any definite cause and they do not accept the theory that the condition is often linked to candidiasis. They point to the following **neurological symptoms** to support their view:

1 Frequent bowel movements especially when the patient is nervous.
2 Bowel movement after meals, especially after breakfast (food stimulates movement of gas which forces the bowels to open)
3 A feeling of fullness in the bowels, even after evacuating stools. There is an urge to go again.
4 Nervousness in going into buildings without toilets, as patients fear accidents. Long car journeys and underground journeys are most feared. People suffering from chronic IBS search for toilets as soon as they enter some premises. They become obsessive, so much so that they avoid crowded places, especially if they are stuck in a queue or a procession.

All these symptoms make physicians think of the psyche. In fact, people lose confidence due to inconsistency of the stools and mucus. Sufferers have so much gas that they have a constant feeling that they want to go to the toilet. The soft stool mass and mucus tend to come out even when releasing gas. It makes them nervous and they fear accidents all the time. Thus IBS becomes a psychological condition.

Before IBS is treated, some basic tests should be carried out to identify and eliminate some common causes of flatulence, abdominal pain and diarrhoea. These tests should include liver function tests, stool tests for microbes and parasites, and blood tests for thyroid problems. Efforts should be made to see if stress may be causing the problem.

Treatment

IBS should be treated with a lot of care. In my opinion every aspect of digestion has to be taken into account to treat it; nothing is to be left to chance. All food should be of moderate quantity and high quality, produced without fertilisers, pesticides and preservatives. You should eat organic foods if possible.

Diet

1 **Fasting** A couple of days of water fast or vegetable broth fast (drink vegetable soup, blended into a purée, as vegetable fibres may irritate the bowels).
2 **Avoid, if stools are frequently loose** roughage as in cereals, bran flakes, spinach, stalks of cauliflower, broccoli, asparagus and cabbage; yeast products, cheese, mushrooms, fried food, curries, citrus fruits, canned products, beer, wine, champagne, chocolates, cakes, cured meats, sausages, fizzy drinks including fizzy water, and butter.

What to eat:
• If constipated – papaya, beetroot, spinach, bananas
• If suffering from diarrhoea – baked or boiled potatoes, overcooked rice, minced meat, yoghurt

3 **Eat slowly** Chew food well. Drink water 30-45 minutes after meals. Rest after lunch. Walk after dinner.

4 **Avoid late dinners** Dinner should be lighter than lunch.

5 **Food should be overcooked** (if stools are soft and there is excessive flatulence).

Specific treatments

1 **Homoeopathy**
2 **Herbal remedies**
   - Peppermint oil capsules, 1–2 per day with meals.
   - Kadu powder (Black Helibore). Soak 1/4 teaspoonful in 1/2 cup of hot water at night. Leave to soak overnight. Drink the water on an empty stomach. This is very bitter in taste.
   - Jwarish Jalinoos (Unani medicine – paste of Galen) Take 1/4 teaspoonful twice daily after meals for 15 days.
   - Papaya tablets – one tablet twice daily for 15 days.
   - **Isabgol** (psyllium husk) is good for constipation. This product came from India where it is a household name. The thin membrane-like husk is rich in fibre. Incidentally, the wheat husk that is separated while making flour is rich in cellulose fibre as well, and is also a powerful laxative. Take 1–2 tablespoons of Isabgol, mix it with a glass of warm water and drink it quickly. The jelly is hard to drink but swallow it quickly. Quickly drink another glass of water afterwards, as the jelly might adhere to the walls of the gullet.
     This has to be drunk at bedtime. The husk is not digested and it is a powerful absorbent. If taken about three hours after dinner, it will absorb undigested food pulp and take it along to the colon. This undigested or semi-digested food mass normally remains in the intestines for hours during the night, especially after a heavy dinner, and causes digestive problems. Sometimes the body generates a second round of digestive activity to destroy this semi-digested food mass. It is like having another meal at night. This is what contributes to weight gain and it is why heavy meals are not recommended at night. Isabgol removes this excess food pulp from the gut.
     Interestingly, Isabgol in water or milk acts as a laxative. In yoghurt, however, it acts as a binding agent and is recommended for diarrhoea.
   - **Senna,** which is widely grown in tropical countries, is a popular laxative. There are several preparations containing this herb and it is a popular drug prescribed by doctors.
   - **Trifola tablets or powder** These contain three Indian herbs – Amla, Bereda and Hidada in equal proportions. This is a mild purgative. It also helps to reduce acid content in the stomach and therefore helps gastritis.

- **Castor oil** This is a very powerful purgative. It irritates the lining of the gut and causes diarrhoea. It is not used as often as it used to be because of its violent effect.
- **Magnesium** This element helps to irritate the bowel lining. It also releases the anal sphincter and facilitates bowel movements.

3 Conventional medicine
- Antidepressants should be taken in extreme cases, when absolutely indicated.
- IBS often causes malabsorption of vitamins and minerals. Calcium and magnesium are poorly absorbed because of irritation of the colon region. Infusions of vitamins and minerals are advisable to replenish the deficiencies. Your physician will tell you which ones are deficient and give you these intravenously.

See your physician for IBS in the following cases:
1 Presence of blood in stools
2 Violent diarrhoea more than six to ten times a day
3 Excessive mucus
4 Fever
5 Colicky abdominal pains occurring very frequently, especially at night
6 Chronic constipation (fewer than two bowel movements per week)
7 Weight loss

Prognosis

The sooner IBS is treated the better. When it becomes chronic, the psychological symptoms become prominent. The diet should be maintained for over six months to consolidate the effect of treatment.

FLATULENCE

Flatulence is a condition whereby there is accumulation and release of gases from the abdomen. It is different from bloating or gas, which is usually in the stomach or small intestines. Flatulence is a condition of the colon or large intestine and the rectum. It is not a disease but a symptom. I'm dealing with it separately because a lot of people suffer from it. Some women are very sensitive about abdominal gas and flatulence for obvious reasons. Clothes become tight and they are conscious about the size of the abdomen.

Some causes of flatulence

1. **Constipation** When the bowel movements are sluggish there is accumulation of gas in the colon. Normally several litres of gas are produced and eliminated. This elimination may take place while walking, bathing, eating or drinking, during bowel movements, and spontaneously at any time. If for some reason this gas is not eliminated, say because of constipation, then there is an excess accumulation of it. Sometimes giardiasis or amoebiasis produce flatulence.

2. **Fermentation** The activity of yeast or fungus on carbohydrates causes fermentation producing alcohol and gas (as in beer).

3. **Putrefication** The action of bacteria on protein or nitrogenous products results in putrefaction or 'rotting'. This produces highly undesirable gases like ammonia and hydrogen sulphide (smell of rotten egg).

4. **Chemical reaction** There are numerous chemical reactions that take place in the intestines. Many of them produce gases which accumulate in the colon.

5. **Excessive consumption of fizzy drinks**
Sometimes flatulence can be excessive, causing discomfort and occasional pain in the abdomen. Excessive flatulence can raise the dome of the diaphragm and cause breathlessness. Sometimes the gas in the colon can push the stomach upwards, enhancing the formation of hiatus hernia. Therefore to treat the symptoms of hiatus hernia (heartburn pain behind the sternum, belching), one has also to treat flatulence. Flatulence can also cause backache when it is chronic and in excess.

Treatment

1. **Change diet** Avoid fizzy drinks, coffee, yeast products, beer, Guinness, champagne, stalks of cauliflower, broccoli and asparagus, roughage as in cereals, radish, chick peas, canned products and sugars.

2. **Eat or drink** beetroot, papaya, carrots (you can juice these), peppermint tea, ginger tea and garlic.

3. **Massage** abdomen with sesame oil in a clockwise direction.

4. **Yogic exercises:** Abdominal pump (E1), Child pose (S1), Turtle pose (M2), Squatting (M1).

Medicines

- **Onion seeds** (Nigella sativa, also known as kolonji) Boil one teaspoonful of seeds in about 250 ml of water for five minutes. Let the mixture stand for five minutes and then drink it.

In some countries in Asia and the Middle East, onion seeds are put into bread. This helps to counter the effects of the gas that the yeast in bread produces. Nigella sativa is a powerful herb with many uses. The Prophet Mohammed wrote about its medicinal properties in the *Hadees*, a practical manual that gives advice on many aspects of daily life. No other religious book in antiquity deals with health and medicine in such detail.

- **Garlic** Chop a pod or two of raw garlic and swallow with water.
- **Fenugreek seeds** Put one teaspoonful of seeds in a glass of warm water and leave to soak overnight. Drink in the morning.
- **Kadu** (Black Helibore) Soak two to three twigs in a cup of hot water at night. Leave to soak overnight. Strain and drink on an empty stomach. This helps to eliminate yeast and other fungus in the gut – sources of flatulence. Moreover, it is a mild purgative and so it helps evacuation of gases.

Prognosis

Habitual flatulence, like constipation, is a very annoying symptom. Sufferers need to follow the regimen of a strict diet as that is the main contributory factor. It is a treatable symptom and it must be treated. Most people neglect it as it doesn't stop them from carrying out their routine activities.

Chapter 20

THE LIFE SUPPORT SYSTEM
Insomnia and sleep disorders

Although physiology divides the body into different systems to make it easier to teach and understand, there is one overall system, the body's life support system, to which all the others belong. Certain conditions affect the whole body outright, and one such is sleep. When the body goes into a deep sleep, pretty well everything shuts down except for the slow chemical processes and basic functions. So sleep disorders directly affect the whole body.

Insomnia has become a major symptom in today's stress-ridden society. In the USA about two-thirds of the population suffer from sleep disorders. Lack of sleep alters people's ability to focus and function normally during the day, and it is for this reason that they approach doctors for help. Students who are tensed before exams can go on for days without sleeping. In fact, many take amphetamines (which have an unusual side-effect of suppressing appetite) to keep themselves awake all night. They don't complain until they are so run down that they cannot function.

Sleep is a very well-documented area in medicine and there are specialists who deal with it separately. The various stages of sleep, the chemicals in the body that induce sleep and the location of the various sleep centres in the brain are very well recorded. Also documented are the various phenomena associated with sleep.

Some may think they are either asleep or awake, but there is much more to it than that. For example, how long should you sleep? Is it quality sleep? It is generally accepted that seven to eight hours of sleep is ideal for adults and yet there are people who sleep much less or much more without any complications in their health whatsoever. Sleep is a habit and varies in different individuals. So it is difficult to define what is normal sleep.

Sleep deficiency

Medicine has drawn a line to divide normal and abnormal sleep by saying that it is abnormal or insufficient when it affects daytime functioning. If lack of sleep leads to lack of concentration, loss of memory, loss of essential reflexes and so on, then this condition is abnormal. Sleep deprivation leads a person to behave in a 'drunken state' where everything is topsy-turvy and it requires a lot of effort to keep their balance.

Drowsiness during the day and a tendency to fall asleep involuntarily is a serious indication of sleep deprivation. In fact, this is a major cause of road traffic accidents. People with serious sleeping problems should not be driving at all. People are banned from driving if they have epilepsy (they can have a fit while driving) or in a drunken state. Chronic lack of sleep should also be a consideration in deciding whether a person should drive or not. So far, legally, this is not an issue, although it is a serious matter as functions like sharp reflexes are essential in driving. Drug companies recognise the seriousness of the matter by indicating on labels that while taking a particular drug one should not drive.

Other aspects of daily life are affected by poor quality sleep, too. General performance at work is affected, people become very irritable, they have serious mood fluctuations and may say tactless or inappropriate things, causing embarrassment to people around them. Therefore lack of sleep has serious behavioural and social implications.

Phases of sleep

The sleep pattern is not continuous throughout the sleeping time. The two phases of sleep are classified as REM (Rapid Eye Movement) and NREM (Non-REM). In the first phase the eyes move rapidly as if seeing things – this is when most of our dreams occur. In the second phase the body is calm and relaxed. These phases alternate every hour or so. On average, 35 per cent of our sleep pattern is of the REM type and 50 per cent of the NREM type, with the remainder of the time being transitional phases between the two. During the NREM sleep pattern various hormones are secreted into the blood to facilitate the various functions in the body. Other hormones such as melatonin are secreted to induce sleep.

Abnormal Sleep (Dissomnias)

1

Insomnia This is lack of sleep for more than three nights per week. An insomnia sufferer sleeps fewer than four hours per night on these days.

2

Sleep apnoea In this condition the breathing stops periodically. For some unknown reason, the upper part of the respiratory tract goes into a spasm and breathing stops for up to two minutes. It always happens to people who are very stressed – perhaps it's nature's way of inducing very deep sleep. However, conventional medicine panics over this and has devised all sorts of apparatus to pump air into the lungs forcefully. I am not sure this is absolutely necessary as even though the breathing stops it kick starts after the pause.

3

Restless leg syndrome Some people with this disorder have an unexplained urge to move their legs. This prevents them from falling asleep. Such people may feel a tingling sensation or a sensation of crawling insects in the leg.

4

Narcolepsy Excessive sleeping characterises this stage. Such people have episodes of uncontrollable urge to asleep.

5

Jet lag This is caused by journeys across time zones. The biological clock is out of rhythm with the daytime period. One is awake when one should be asleep and vice versa.

Insomnia

Amongst these five groups, insomnia is the most common form of sleep disorder. It is divided into four categories:

- difficulty in falling asleep
- frequent awakening at night

- early morning awakening (between 3 and 4 a.m.)
- persistent sleepiness despite adequate sleep.

It must be noted that 'feeling tired', 'chronically fatigued' and 'constantly lethargic' are not necessarily signs of sleeping disorder. These conditions could be triggered by problems such as chronic fatigue syndrome, premenstrual syndrome, osteoporosis or anaemia. It is important to differentiate between tiredness caused by lack of sleep and tiredness resulting from other ailments.

A poor sleeping habit is developed by stressful events. These habits may continue even though the stress may not be persistent. Some people are so agitated by not being able to sleep that they toss and turn and curse themselves. They become so frustrated that they cannot sleep. Such people arouse themselves with their own thoughts.

Changes in the sleeping environment can cause sleep disturbances. A different hotel, unfamiliar surroundings, the presence of a snoring partner, street sounds, or uncontrolled room temperature (either too hot or cold) can cause sleeping disturbances. As can large meals, late dinners, excessive exercises and hot baths before sleeping.

Certain drugs and alcohol cause sleep disorders. Caffeine is the most common cause of insomnia in sensitive people. The muscles tense up and such people are unable to relax. Many people are surprised when they are told about this. Similarly alcohol and nicotine (smoking) can interfere with sleep. Although alcohol increases drowsiness and helps a person to fall asleep in the initial phase, it disturbs people and later on interferes with their sleep. Drugs such as cocaine and ecstasy excite the brain and arouse the body to keep going without sleep.

At high altitude people have insomnia due to lack of oxygen and increased carbon dioxide in the blood. This alters the pattern of breathing. First the breathing gets heavier and then it stops suddenly for a few seconds, only to restart with a gradual increase. This disturbs sleep. Being a keen trekker in the Himalayas, I am familiar with this breathing pattern, which is known as Cheyne-Stokes breathing. A similar pattern can be observed in aeroplanes. I suspect the oxygen concentration in these planes is deliberately lowered at night or sleep time to economise on its use.

Parasomnias

This term refers to behavioural disorders during sleep which have little or no effect on the depth of the sleep or daytime performance.

1

Sleepwalking (somnambulism) Sleepwalkers can carry out simple to complex activities while still in a deep sleep. They may walk, even urinate, wherever they want to. This disorder is common in children and adolescents.

2

Sleep terror Children and adolescents have nightmares and panic attacks. They scream, sweat profusely, breathe frequently and have palpitation.

3

Grinding teeth in sleep (bruxism) Some people grind their teeth in their sleep and sometimes the noise is so loud that a partner can be woken up.

4

Bedwetting Before the age of five or six, children very often wet their bed. This is considered normal but if it continues beyond that age it is considered to be a medical problem.

Other sleep disorders

1

Psychiatric diseases Schizophrenia, depression, mania, etc., cause sleep disturbances. In fact, one of the first symptoms of these illnesses is loss of sleep.

2

Neurological diseases These include stroke, Parkinson's disease, epilepsy and migraine.

3

Diseases that cause painful conditions Pain from a 'slipped disc', rheumatoid arthritis, heartburn or irritable bowel syndrome, for example, can arouse the person very easily. In diabetes or prostate enlargement people often need to go to the toilet at night, thus disturbing their sleep. Asthma and bronchitis are common causes of disturbed sleep, as attacks normally come at around 4 a.m.

4

Unusual sleeping patterns Some people come home from work, sit before the TV and fall asleep. Such people often stay up at night till late. Others cannot sleep until the early hours of the morning. Shift workers who work at night burn up their night fuel and are often unable to rest adequately. Continuous night shifts may alter the sleeping pattern. During the day it is not easy to find the right sleeping environment as there is always light, noise, phone calls, visitors, and so on.

Thus we can see that something as simple as sleep has many ramifications. Although under normal circumstances one can sleep well, the introduction of stress or some disturbance causes everything to go wrong. In an urban society with all its stress, electronic gadgets, late-night entertainment, frequent travelling and cramped premises, it is increasingly difficult to find an ideal situation for sound sleep. It is not surprising, then, that sleep is such a major problem in medicine. Sleeping tablets, whether natural or chemical, are perhaps one of the top five best-selling drugs. People take them and adapt to them, and the tablets become a decreasingly effective habit. So they take more.

Treatment of insomnia

Diet

Avoid alcohol at night and coffee at any time. **Also avoid** eating or drinking anything that may cause acid, gas or excessive flatulence because abdominal discomfort and the goings-on in the intestines send wakeful messages to the brain. These products include very spicy curries, chickpeas, cold milk, fizzy drinks, beer or bitter, mushrooms, canned products, yeast products, MSG (Chinese food) and citrus fruits. If you are constipated make sure it is properly treated. The abdominal gas may cause cramps and hiatus hernia which often wake people up in the middle of the night. Do not eat heavy dinners, as the digestive process may cause heartburn, burping, rumbling stomach and so on. Avoid dessert at dinner time and do not drink sweet, hot drinks (chocolate, cocoa, tea) at bedtime. These may initially be comforting but the sugar agitates the brain, perhaps by giving fuel to it when it needs to be calmed down.

Other lifestyle changes

- Do not watch disturbing movies or hold serious late-night conversations (finish business and stressful discussions during the day).
- Walk for ten minutes (even inside the house) after dinner.
- Cut down or stop smoking, because nicotine interferes with sleep. Smoking may temporarily relax you but excessive nicotine irritates the brain.
- Drink water before going to bed or keep water near your bed. People who are stressed or do heavy physical work during the day have a demand for fluids even at night. When you are dehydrated, your pulse rate goes up and this is a major cause of the 'anxiety' at night which disturbs many people. If such a thing happens drink a little water.

The bedroom and sleeping positions

1

Use the bedroom exclusively for sleeping if possible. Once you are in the bedroom you then know that you are to sleep and not work, eat or watch television.

2

The bed and pillows should be comfortable. A firm bed with low pillows is good. Uncomfortable beds are often a big problem. Thick or multiple pillows often make the neck stiff and cause great discomfort at night. Moreover they might impair the flow of blood to the brain and cause sleep disturbances. If you travel a lot, carry your own pillow or ask the hotel to arrange for one that will suit you. If you have asthma or hiatus hernia you may feel more comfortable using more than one pillow, but keep them to the minimum you really need.

If you are in the habit of sleeping on your side, get yourself a soft pillow, the thickness of which should be equal to the length of your shoulder (between the neck and the actual shoulder joint). When lying on it the soft pillow will shrink a little and give your neck a comfortable position to rest sideways.

If you prefer to sleep on your back, the thickness of the soft pillow should be such that the head is slightly raised and the chin level with the chest. This creates an ideal condition for the blood supply to the brain during sleep.

If you move around at night and sleep both on your sides and on your back, then use the pillow you would use to sleep on your back and bunch it up to create an extra thickness that would allow you to sleep on your side.

Sleeping on the stomach is not good for the neck. The sooner you eliminate this habit the better. To change it is not difficult. After a couple of nights of slight discomfort you will soon be used to a new position.

3

Get rid of electronic gadgets from your bedroom because they emit radiation that affects the brain. This includes computers, music systems and TVs (especially when the clock flickers at night). Get rid of clocks that tick. Draw the curtains. If your street is noisy keep the windows shut.

4

Make sure the blankets and duvets you use do not make you feel uncomfortable at night (neither too hot nor too cold). Remember that during sleep the system that regulates your body temperature (thermo-regulation) is switched off and so the body can get hot or cold very easily depending on the outside temperature. This can actually make you uncomfortable and disturb your sleep. The room temperature also matters and therefore you should keep it at around 20–22 ºC. This is ideal for sleeping with a light blanket, which will help to trap your body heat to a comfortable level. Too warm a temperature may dehydrate you.

5

Feng-Shui (Chinese) and Vatsu Shastra (the Indian equivalent) are two art forms of architecture and landscaping which take into consideration nature and the natural phenomena that affect our mind and body. The planning of houses and the environment within takes these into consideration. According to this art form, one should sleep with the head pointing north. Perhaps these ancients took the earth's magnetic field into consideration. (In Islam even the bodies are buried with the head pointing northwards in the Northern hemisphere.)

6

Avoid wearing tight clothes. Loose fitting clothes are much better.

7

Do not take hot baths just before going to bed. The blood vessels dilate and invigorate the mind and body. This may be detrimental to sound sleep.

8

If your partner snores, use ear plugs or sleep in a different room. This second option is a harsh one but many a family has broken down because of snoring problems. It is something that a judge might consider in order to decide on the grounds for divorce.

Other therapies

There is no universal remedy for sleep that will suit everybody. The causes of insomnia are many and that is why it is considered to be multifactorial. You'll have to try various options and select the one that suits you. Do the **Regimen Therapy** along with it. If a remedy you use regularly loses its effectiveness, change it. Here are some suggestions.

1

Massage Husbands and wives should massage each other's neck and shoulders for five to ten minutes before going to sleep. Most of the physical and mental stress accumulates in the neck and shoulder area. I suggest the most appropriate oil is two tablespoons of base oil with six drops each of lavender and camomile oils added. This massage releases the tension and improves blood flow to the brain stem where most of the sleep-regulating systems are located. Moreover, it has a very pleasant effect on the mind.

2

Exercises Before going to bed, the following five-minute exercise programme is advisable: Half cobra (P2), Turtle (M2), Semi-bridge (S3), Spinal twist (M3), Head roll (E3) followed by Shavasana (S4) on the bed (see pages 66–73).

The Shavasana is a powerful yogic mental exercise, it induces sleep and calms the mind. The sleep becomes better quality. If it is done every day, it will condition the body to sleep. If you wake up in the middle of the night, do the Shavasana and it will help you to get back to sleep.

3

Acupuncture induces good sleep. A session of acupuncture can help people to recover from jetlag syndrome if done under an experienced practitioner. When there is a prolonged period of stress, acupuncture helps mitigate it. Some points (stomach 36, heart 7) can induce sleep instantly.

4

Homoeopathy helps to relieve stress and to restore sleep. An old homoeopath in India once gave me a recipe for sleep:

Two tablets of Nux Vomica 200 on the tongue at bedtime, followed five minutes later by two tablets of Belladonna 30 on the tongue. I use this combination very often. Nux Vomica is said to relax muscle tension, whereas Belladonna removes wild thoughts in the head. The combination seems to be ideal for insomnia due to stress and tension. You can repeat this combination when you wake up in the middle of the night with anxiety and panic. Drink a glass of water to relieve dehydration, if there is any, and take these homoeopathic remedies.

5

Herbal remedies You will have to try out these remedies to see which one, either in single dose or in combination, suits you. Consult your doctor or herbalist for guidance.

- Valeriana drops – 10–15 drops in 1/4 cup of water at bedtime
- Passiflora – tablets or 10–15 drops in 1/4 cup of water at bedtime
- Avena sativa – 10–15 drops in 1/4 cup of water at bedtime
- Ayurvedic remedy: 1/2 teaspoonful each of powdered Shankh Puspi and Jatamansi to be boiled in a glass of water for five minutes. Strain, cool and drink at bedtime.
- Brahmi oil massage of the head at bedtime.

6

Meditation This will help you to switch off very quickly and help induce good sleep.

7

Conventional medicine If the stress level is high and none of the above helps then consult your doctor for sleeping pills, but be warned – they are addictive.

Treatment for other sleep disorders

Bed-wetting (children)

- **Diet** The evening meal should be eaten as early as possible. Avoid soups, juices, soft drinks, salty snacks, sweets, deep-fried food, spicy food and jams and marmalades. Some of these foods tend to be dehydrating and will make the child want more water. The intake of water should be reduced after 4 p.m. although it is important to drink normally earlier in the day.
- **Massage** Massage the neck, spine and lower abdomen at bedtime.
- **Homoeopathic medicine** and **acupuncture** can also be effective.

Bruxism

- Massage the neck, jaws, temples and the joint of the jaw just in front of the ears at bedtime.
- Do the breathing and relaxation exercise described on pages 68–69.

- Use a low pillow.
- Try using a mouth guard.
- See your dentist if none of these remedies work.

Narcolepsy

- Deep-tissue massage, especially of the neck area.
- Walk in the fresh air for an hour every day.
- Avoid alcohol.
- Do regular yoga exercises (the entire range described on pages 64–73).

Restless leg syndrome

- Massage at bedtime.
- Relaxation exercises e.g. Shavasana (S4) on page 68.

Sleep apnoea

- Breathing exercises (page 64).
- Relaxation exercises e.g. Shavasana (S4) on page 68.
- Deep massage of the neck and jaws.
- Use a low pillow.

Sleep terrors and sleepwalking

- Massage the neck and spine at bedtime every night for a month.
- Children should avoid caffeine and sugars (e.g. sweets, chocolate) at bedtime and drink water immediately before going to bed to avoid dehydration.
- They should avoid watching TV or playing computer games, etc., at bedtime.

Chapter 21

THE IMMUNE SYSTEM
Fungal infections

THE IMMUNE SYSTEM

The immune system, an important part of our sanogenetic power (see pages 8–9), consists of the lymphatic system, bone marrow, spleen and, to a certain extent, the liver. Its main function is to defend the body from bacteria, viruses, fungi and allergens (dust, pollen, foodstuffs, etc.) that might enter the body. It is the defence ministry of the body with its military forces to fight invaders (the antibodies), intelligence-gathering service (the lymph nodes), and armament factory (bone marrow, spleen, liver, thyroid gland, etc.). Bacteria and viruses are living material so they are attacked with antibodies that block their activities and destroy them. They could also be captured by white blood cells (phagocytes) and eaten up. Allergens (dust, pollen, etc.) are non-living and therefore the only way to deal with them is to throw them out of the body by an allergic reaction (runny nose, diarrhoea, skin rash, hives, etc.).

All these reactions are carried out by the immune system. It recognises enemy agents and deals with them. Sometimes, however, it makes mistakes. Certain tissues, such as joint membranes or connective tissue, or the tissue of the kidneys or lungs, often change their structure due to an infection or some other process. Now these tissues, because of their transformation, become alien to the body. The immunological detectives (the 'intelligence agency') find them and treat them like traitors. Suddenly the immune system produces an aggressive reaction with antibodies and attacks the transformed tissue. This is what happens in auto-immune diseases like lupus and rheumatoid arthritis. In rheumatoid arthritis, for example, joint membranes fall victim to the body's powerful immune system and serious inflammation and deformation takes place.

Adaptation

The immune system is one of the more outstanding systems of adaptation in our body. While it will constantly adapt to new conditions and diseases to give us protection, if those conditions are not supportive to it (such as when drugs are ingested which interfere with its activities), then it is likely to adapt in a negative way by ceasing its operations and even suppressing part of its defences altogether. For example, taking steroids usually suppresses the secretion of the body's own natural steroids and, if prolonged, the glands themselves can become permanently deactivated. An outstanding example of such a negative response is the emergence of fungal infections, which has resulted from the widespread and irresponsible misuse of antibiotics.

Antibiotics: the problem

Fungal infections are more common now than they used to be. Before the use of antibiotics, fungal infections in the body occurred rarely. Antibiotics, which came into general use with the discovery of penicillin in the 1940s, are fungal products, derived from a mycelium or mould, whose toxins suppress the growth of bacteria. When antibiotics were first developed, it seemed that the battle against bacterial infection was over, and medicine had won. Penicillin and its derivatives were used indiscriminately for decades to treat everything that gave the slightest hint of involving an infection.

Several problems have arisen from this. The bacteria mutated and became resistant to antibiotics. New forms of antibiotic were developed to combat this, but the bacteria continued to mutate too. Today, bacterial infections such as MRSA, which are found so widely in hospitals, are resistant to most conventional antibiotics.

In nature there was a balance between the bacterium, the fungus and the virus, the three leading agents that invade the body and live as parasites. By beating bacteria hard with antibiotics for so many years, we have ruined the balance. The immune system no longer needs to fight off bacteria, because antibiotics do the job for it. The result is a weakening of the immune system overall, so that when the body is attacked by fungal or viral infections it takes much longer for the body to fight them off.

Nowadays classical bacterial infections, such as pneumonia, streptococcal throat infections, meningococcal meningitis and bacterial dysentery, are rare. What we see more often is viral pneumonia, gastric flu, viral meningitis and so on, against which antibiotics are useless (although some doctors still prescribe them). We are also seeing an increase in fungal infections.

FUNGAL INFECTION

The problem with fungus is that it thrives outside the boundaries of the body. Hair, nails, gut, skin, vagina, mouth and ears are all at the fringes of the body. They are in contact with the atmosphere (even the gut is a long tube with two openings). That is why the body cannot organise an effective defence against the fungus. It would have to fire 'antibodies' into the atmosphere like rockets. Therefore fungal infections have a huge advantage – they can thrive without the body being able to do anything constructive against them. Bacteria and viruses circulate in the blood and thrive inside the body. Fungi, if they enter the body, go undercover by coating themselves with a hard spore, which the body's detectives and security guards (the immune system) cannot identify.

Fungal infections can be conquered by one method only – making the body strong and resistant once again so that fungal infections do not get a chance to survive, even on its surface. That is a mammoth task, especially when doctors have abused the body with antibiotics for so long.

Main types of fungal infection:

1

Yeast overgrowth and candidiasis in the gut This is characterised by bloating, abdominal pain, fatigue and toxic reactions such as headache and nausea.

2

Thrush or fungal infection of the mouth This is characterised by mouth ulcers which can be very painful.

3

Vaginal thrush Candida albicans is the main fungus involved in this type of overgrowth in the vagina. White yoghurt-like discharge with local itching and irritation are the main symptoms.

4

Fungal infection of the nails It is generally the toenails that are affected by fungus. The nails get deformed and brittle.

5

Fungal infection of the hair follicles This causes loss of hair in patches. It is called **alopecia areata** when a round patch of the scalp or beard has no hair. The fungus attacks the follicles and the hair becomes weak and falls off.

6

Fungal infection of the skin Certain types of fungus can attack the skin. This causes depigmentation in areas of the skin. This condition is often associated with swimming in hot places.

7

Athlete's foot

Treatment

You should follow the **Regimen Therapy** consisting of a strict antifungal diet, massages of the neck and shoulder area and the general yoga exercises detailed on pages 64–73, to help the body to build up its sanogenetic powers. This makes the body less susceptible to fungal, bacterial and viral infections. Boosting your general health is particularly important if you have fungal infections of the nails or hair because these conditions are difficult to treat in any other way. The tissues in these areas are basically 'dead' tissues, with no link to the lymphatic or circulatory systems, and therefore medicines taken by mouth cannot reach them. Fungal creams are washed away too easily and cannot penetrate to the core of the cuticles, while more corrosive applications cause more damage to the tissues.

Diet

Avoid all yeast products (bread, pizza, pitta bread, Marmite, canned products, gravy sauce in bottles), sugars, citrus fruits, alcohol, coffee and mushrooms. You should also avoid smoked fish and meat, hard cheeses, grapes and dried fruit because these products have microscopic coatings of mould.

Combine protein with vegetables and restrict carbohydrates to a minimum. Eat a small amount of pasta, rice or potato, but combine chicken or fish with vegetables. Sometimes **fasting** for two to three days with water, honey and drops of lemon juice is very beneficial. It is also advisable to go on a **vegetarian diet** of vegetables, vegetable soup, some rice or yeast-free bread for about two weeks.

Medicines

1

Kadu (Black Helibore) Soak two to three twigs or ¼ teaspoon of powder in a cup of hot water at night. Leave to soak overnight. Strain and drink in the morning. You will need to continue this treatment for two to three months.

2

Caprylic acid in capsules. Consult physician.

3

Grape seed oil in capsules. Consult physician.

4

Infusions of vitamin C and B12 intravenously help to boost the body.

5

Nystatin (conventional antifungal preparation). This should be taken when the fungal infection is very severe (for example vaginal or oral thrush causing severe discomfort). Consult your physician for this.

6

Acidophyllus with Bifido capsules

Topical applications

A number of antifungal creams are available. Consult your doctor if the fungal infection is severe.

1

For athlete's foot mix the following in a bottle:
  2 parts pine oil
  4 parts neem oil
  2 parts eucalyptus oil
  2 parts kolonji oil

Wet pieces of cotton wool with this mixture of oils and place them between the toes. Remove after 20 minutes and keep the area dry.

2

For fungal infection of the skin soak cotton wool in fresh lime juice and apply to the affected area, twice daily for two to four weeks.

3

For vaginal thrush Soak cotton wool or a tampon in live yoghurt and insert into the vagina. Leave for a few hours.

4

For alopecia areata rub kolonji oil (Nigella Sativa) onto the affected area. (A Hakim or traditional Unani physician once told me of an interesting recipe. He said finely powdered ivory was mixed with rarefied butter (ghee) and applied on the affected area daily for a month.)

5

For ringworm or fungal infection of the skin in the groin region, apply sulphur powder mixed with a 2 per cent salicylic-acid-based cream to the affected area, once a day for a week.

Prognosis

Some fungal infections, such as alopecia areata and fungal infections of the nails, are more difficult to treat than others, but all fungal infections should be treated early, when they first appear. The longer they remain on the body surface, the more powerful they become.

Chapter 22

T HE TWO GREAT KILLERS
Cancer and heart disease

Though killer diseases are not part of a system as such, some mention of such an important category is appropriate here, especially when critical steps can be taken in integrated medicine to mitigate or prevent them, as in the case of cancer or heart disease.

CANCER

The integrated medical approach to cancer is the subject of a book in itself, so what follows should be regarded as no more than guidelines. Cancer is a multifactorial disease, as no single, common causative factor has been found. Certain substances have carcinogenic effects, but it requires particular situations, like prolonged stress, for the immune system to break down. For decades scientists have been trying to find a definitive answer to the question 'What causes cancer?' and have failed miserably. What is true for one person may not be true for another. Although stress is a common aggravating factor, its direct causative effect cannot be established. People respond differently to stress – some may have high blood pressure, some psoriasis, others mental illnesses, and some cancer.

My approach is that when one does not know what causes an ailment it is best to look after the body and mind to maintain an equilibrium. This is the optimum approach, as we have generally accepted in this book that in 80 per cent of cases the body's sanogenetic powers can manage on their own. If the right conditions are laid down then the body correctly balances by itself and restores health.

In the case of cancer, a strict **Regimen Therapy** with powerful dietary and stress management elements can slow down processes that aggravate cancer (see the summary on page 45). Rest is especially important, as is meditation. Learn simple meditation techniques from a qualified teacher and practise regularly. If you can't find an instructor, practise the yogic Shavasana, also a powerful relaxation technique. These techniques calm your nervous system and slow down the body. This can help the body to slow down the erratic division of cancer cells.

Treatment

Chemotherapy and radiotherapy

There is no doubt that conventional chemotherapy can sometimes suppress the growth of cancer cells, but that comes at a heavy cost. The side-effects of chemotherapeutic drugs are extreme. They damage the liver, kidneys, and other healthy tissues, and have a devastating effect on the immune system. If these side-effects were not there, then perhaps chemotherapy would be the best option. Scientists are working on drugs that would target only cancer cells and produce minimum side-effects. Such an approach will help the body tremendously.

Radiotherapy and surgery target the cancer growths directly if they are large enough. But while some growth areas can be detected by scanning techniques, there are others that are too small to be identified. Moreover, the cancer cells can travel to different parts of the body and start new 'colonies'. These are known as secondaries or metastatic cancer areas. Therefore both radiotherapy and surgery are useless in eradicating cancer completely.

Complementary therapies

New treatments for cancer include a wide range of traditional and high-tech medicines. Fasting, coffee enemas, naturopathy, healing, yoga, meditation, Infusions of vitamins and minerals, injections of apricot seed extracts, Chinese herbal medicines, various herbal preparations claimed to have anti-cancer properties, magnetic therapy, and ozone/oxygen therapy are all available. Therapies banned in the USA are available in clinics just over the border in Mexico. These clinics have offered hope to many sufferers, as many patients have gone into remission. What causes the remission is not important in Mexico, so long as the drugs do not have side-effects and patients benefit from them. People have the right to live and they also have the right to choose how to live, within the general guidelines of the law.

In their quest to help their patients some doctors have applied many of these treatments at the same time, hoping that something will work. As one doctor said, 'Throw everything on the wall and hope that something will stick. If patients survive then it is fine, but if they don't one may reasonably assume there was no hope for them anyway.' I am not sure I can agree with this approach, unless of course all other avenues are closed.

The integrated medicine approach

At the Integrated Medical Centre we work hand-in-hand with conventional medical doctors, liaising with them throughout the treatment whenever possible. Sometimes our patients opt for oncologists who are sympathetic to complementary and traditional medicine. This makes our task easier because the dose of the chemotherapeutic drug does not have to be so high, nor the duration of treatment so long as is recommended in the pharmaceutical guidelines if other therapies have a synergistic effect. For example, if a reduced dose of chemotherapy is supported by diet, relaxation techniques, massages, infusions of vitamin C, magnesium, calcium and selenium, and yoga, then the chances are there will be fewer side-effects. Our experience shows that such patients do not suffer from any side-effects of chemotherapy and they can go through the entire course without fatigue, loss of appetite, nausea and so on.

In between the chemotherapy sessions, we suggest that patients go on a fruit and vegetable diet for a couple of days, followed by a nourishing diet as described on page 50. This ensures quicker elimination of the toxic chemicals.

Once the chemotherapy is over, a patient usually goes through a regime of occasional fasting followed by a strict diet. The aim is to combine detoxifying with building up the body. There is no point, I feel, in starving the body of food by going on a fruit-juice-only diet. After chemotherapy the body is under great stress and it tries very hard to cope. To starve it completely, especially when the appetite is low anyway, is not a sensible thing. The body needs enzymes and proteins to carry out biochemical processes. A toxic liver is in no condition to process any food for a few days so it is best to fast or stay on juices. As soon as the liver throws out the toxins, nourishment should immediately be given through food.

A strict vegetarian diet is not a solution either. All toxins are eliminated from the body with the help of proteins. All enzymes are proteins and therefore protein should be an essential part of the diet. Starving the body beyond its capacity does not help cancer in the long run, though it may in the initial phase. The principle of 'starve the body, starve the cancer' is not a very sensible one. In reality things don't work that way. You need to feed the body correctly to arouse the sanogenetic powers to function.

Prognosis

The prognosis of cancer has improved in recent years. There are growing reports of cancer survivors and people who have gone into long remission. When I was practising in India I had over a hundred cancer patients who exceeded normal survival expectations, some by many years. At the Integrated Medical Centre we have a couple of dozen patients who have gone into remission and are comfortable. Some have been symptom-free for over five years, the deadline to be regarded as a cure, and we sincerely hope they do not go back to their active stage again. Such sporadic cases of success cannot be considered as anecdotal anymore, however sceptical conventional medical science and the institutions might be.

People are becoming more aware of cancer and its complications. Regular check-ups have led to early detection. The sooner it is treated, the better the results. This has been one of the factors that has led to the success of cancer treatment. The other major factor is that people are changing their lifestyle after the shock of discovery of cancer. This self-imposed lifestyle programme is a form of Regimen Therapy.

Cancer treatment is expensive. This hurts if you have to pay from your own resources. Chemotherapy is very expensive but if you were to try the different non-conventional therapies mentioned above it would not be cheap either. It is better for people to opt for the less expensive Regimen Therapy as it is based on self-help.

Most doctors know that chemotherapy does not really help to cure cancer. It is only used to buy time, at great cost to the patient's health. There may be a period of remission after the first course of chemotherapy and people get false hope. The disease normally returns with a vengeance, especially if no lifestyle changes are carried out in the interim period. Second time around the disease usually spreads very fast and even chemotherapy has little or no effect.

Regimen Therapy offers two approaches. Used as an alternative, the remissions achieved are comparable with those obtained by conventional medicine. As a complement to chemotherapy, it results in substantial improvements in the quality of life and probably the best overall prospects of extended remission.

HEART DISEASE

Heart disease is one of the major killers in the West. The ironic thing about it is that it is largely preventable. It is a man-made disease, something that people inflict upon themselves. Several studies have shown that diet, stress, obesity, diabetes, lack of exercise, high blood pressure, smoking and alcohol abuse increase the risk of heart attacks. In the UK, studies done on ethnic groups show that people from Southern Asia (Indians, Pakistanis) are at highest risk of heart disease. The use of ghee (clarified butter) in cooking, fried food, rich curries (curries are generally overcooked, over-greased and overspiced foods), lack of exercise, alcohol abuse, diabetes and smoking are all contributory factors.

Another common denominator is the genetic factor. Heart disease has a strong genetic link. It simply runs in the family.

There are several types of heart disease, and I will cover the two main ones – ischaemic heart disease (angina, heart attack) and heart failure – with just a word about cardiac arrest.

Ischaemic heart disease

Ischaemic heart disease (*isch* – lack of; *haemia* – blood) is a condition in which the heart muscles do not get enough blood. The heart is a muscular organ that contracts and expands throughout your life span. The heartbeat is the main parameter of life. So long as the heart beats you are alive.

Heart muscles have a network of numerous blood vessels, because they need oxygen and glucose all the time and must eliminate waste (carbon dioxide) all the time. Blood flow to the heart muscles is of paramount importance. The slightest reduction in blood supply can make the muscles falter. As in a jet engine, the fuel supply must be constant. A reduction in the blood supply (ischaemia) causes erratic behaviour of the heart muscles, which produces a range of potentially lethal complications. For example, weakened heart muscles may not contract and the heart will stop.

The blood flows to the heart muscles via the arteries of the heart. When plaque is formed in them there is a reduced flow of blood. Any form of exertion (walking, climbing stairs, stress) makes the heart beat faster and the demand for blood increases. However, the supply is poor. This causes lactic acid to be formed (because sugar does not have enough oxygen to convert itself to the final products – carbon dioxide and water – but only to an intermediary product, lactic acid). The lactic acid causes the heart muscles to ache. This ache is called angina pectoris – pain in the chest. Similar aches or cramps can be felt in calf muscles when one runs a lot.

When the chest pains start you have to stop and take a breath to let it pass. If it doesn't stop, then you have to take a pill under your tongue (the veins under the tongue can absorb certain medicines quickly and transfer them to the heart) to dilate the blood vessels, thus improving the blood flow.

Sometimes the furring of the arteries is so great that there is a potential risk of some plaque ripping off and blocking a small blood vessel, cutting off blood supply to an entire region of the heart. This can also result from clot formation in the small arteries of the heart. Once a section of the heart loses blood supply, this part fails to function. The heart cannot pump efficiently and this is what a heart attack is. The body begins to panic, the circulation to the entire body gets cut off and the victim can even collapse unconscious. There is chest pain, cold sweat, anxiety, numbness in the hands and feet, and breathlessness. Unless medical help is available immediately (oxygen is given, together with drugs to dissolve clots or thin the blood, or drugs to dilate blood vessels), the heart may stop (cardiac arrest). The complications of a heart attack depend solely on whether the heart continues to beat or not.

Fortunately, heart muscles can repair themselves and function normally again, although scar tissue is formed where the muscles have been damaged. Depending on the percentage of blockage, people can be treated conservatively with drugs and lifestyle changes, or surgically by ballooning (dilating the artery with a 'balloon'), stenting (a small tube is inserted in the plaqued artery) and bypassing (an arterial graft from a piece of vein in the leg bypasses the clotted or narrowed area). A surgical solution is best for the heart as new channels are created to replace or bypass the old blocked one.

Modern techniques can be used to identify the degree of occlusion (by plaque formation) in the arteries of the heart. Electrocardiograph, ultrasound and angiogram (injecting a dye and then photographing the extent of loss of blood flow) are used to identify the damage to heart muscles and the areas of narrowing of blood vessels. Then the decision is made to treat with either drugs or surgery. Usually surgeons wait till the narrowing of the arteries is over 65 per cent. Just like all other replacement surgeries, you have to wait for advanced degeneration before they will operate. That is the paradox – you live with a dagger hanging over your head, hoping that the thread won't snap. The risk of a heart attack is always there, however small it may be, and not enough stress is placed on preventive measures. Most people continue with their old lifestyle so that the narrowing crosses the dangerous 65 per cent level. Only the fortunate ones can have an angiogram every now and then to see the stage they have reached and if they qualify for ballooning or surgery. The majority of people end up having further episodes of heart attacks while they wait. This risk is being reduced by the introduction of new and cost-effective technology. Frequent screenings help to identify the severity of the problem.

Reducing the risks

If, at this crucial stage, patients can be persuaded to change their regimen or lifestyle by altering their diet and doing exercises, the risk is reduced to a minimum. Somehow not enough is being done to combat the biggest killer in modern society. It is almost as if someone, somewhere, is keeping the problem unsolved on purpose — as if to support an entire industry that manufactures medicines that keep the machinery going, or the profession that deals with it.

Prevention of heart disease is a simple method but one that requires a lot of discipline. The crucial thing is lifestyle change and that is something most people fail to do. They bring this potentially lethal disease on to themselves. The following list highlights the key changes that are needed.

1

Weight loss Obesity increases the risk of heart disease. It leads to high blood pressure and plaque formation in the arteries.

2

Reducing the cholesterol level in the blood reduces the risk of plaque formation.

3

Controlling diabetes and hypertension This reduces the risk of plaque formation in the arteries.

4

Quitting smoking Smoking increases the plaque formation in the arteries. It also reduces the oxygenation of blood in the lungs. That means less oxygen reaches the heart muscles.

5

Stress management, to reduce blood pressure and control the factors that increase the load on the heart. The function of the heart is closely related to emotions. That is why the ancient people used to think that the heart and not the brain was the seat of emotions. All grief, anxiety, worry and so on are felt through the heart, because the rhythm of the heart changes with psychological movements.

6

Exercises They say exercise is the best remedy for the heart. Being a muscular organ it does not like to be idle. Carry out the general daily exercises detailed on pages 64–73.

If one takes these preventive measures, especially after 40 years of age, the risk of heart disease is minimised. **Regimen Therapy** includes most of the preventive measures for heart disease.

Most people who have a heart attack are shocked because they come very close to death. That is why, when people get any kind of pain in the chest and left arm, they get really nervous with symptoms of sweating and fright. They are only relieved when the diagnosis turns out to be neurological (nerve) pain or muscle ache.

Once the emergency situation of a heart attack is over, most patients do exactly as they are told: fat-free diet, no smoking, no drinking and plenty of exercise. They even promise to cut down on their stress level by going slow. A significant proportion of people do that. Having a heart attack takes a lot out of them. Unfortunately, most people cannot fight the temptation of 'good' living. Many of the things they are asked to avoid are addictive – cigarettes, alcohol, fatty foods, chocolates . . . Regrettably physicians do not place much emphasis on this part and leave the patients to get over their habits and addictions. Family members panic and keep nagging the patients to do this or that, which is counter-productive, at least for addiction.

I think cardiologists and mental health care workers should place special emphasis on the preventive aspect of management of heart disease, and governments should give the necessary administrative support. This will see a drop in queues for heart surgery and cut the cost of the healthcare budget drastically (even a fraction of $200 billion is a lot of money). After all, the people have to take some responsibility for their health. Those who lead a decadent lifestyle acquire all the negative elements of heart disease, and when they are sick they want the healthcare system to be responsible for it. Whose fault is it? One can understand the people who are victims of their family genetic structure, or who have high cholesterol or high blood pressure despite their efforts to diet and relax. These people, however, are only a small fraction of the large numbers who get heart disease.

Managing ischaemic heart disease:

Diet

In ischaemic heart disease the diet is the most important factor. The main reason why people go for the wrong foods is the taste and variety. If they tell themselves that for a year or two they will follow a strict diet regime to reverse the process that leads to heart disease, then they can use the principle of moderation and variety to lead an almost 'normal' life. Whatever the reasoning, heart patients have to follow a strict regime for a year or so before they can qualify for a slightly varied lifestyle. One must remember that heart disease is preventable and manageable.

Avoid: Coffee (constricts blood vessels – not good), fats and oils (butter, excessive oil), cheese (fat content is high), excess salt (bad for blood pressure), red meat (beef, lamb, pork – high fat content), shellfish (high in cholesterol), canned or preserved foods (excess salt), gravy sauce (high salt content), cured meats (salt content), alcohol (helps absorption of fats), chocolates, cakes and sweets (promotes weight gain).

It is best to use common sense in selecting the food products. Eating at home is very sensible as you have full control of what you eat. In restaurants and at other people's houses you eat what you are served. That is not the right thing for heart patients.

A diet that is good for the heart does not have to be boring. If you vary your menu and use different herbs and spices to flavour the food, then there is less problem. You can easily go on the total fat-free diet for a year after ischaemic heart disease is diagnosed. Use natural fats in fish and chicken and plenty of garnish or spices to flavour the food. Since food is the most important factor in ischaemic heart disease, much emphasis has to be given to this aspect.

Fasting

Fasting is a good method of keeping a check on all the dietary factors that promote heart disease. Moreover, it helps to control blood pressure and creates a certain amount of calmness which helps the heart. The most beneficial part of fasting is the building up of the willpower. By refraining from food, controlling your desire to eat, fighting certain temptations to eat and creating a certain discipline in your life, you create an ideal situation to fight any chronic ailment, whether it be heart disease or something else. You should fast once a week and, if possible, do a three-day fast every six months.

If possible, you should do a total fast apart from water, or water with 1/2 teaspoon of honey and 5 drops of lemon juice added per glass. Alternatively, you should have a fruit and soup day, and drink juices or water. Tangerines, satsumas and oranges that are not very sour (non-hybrid and non GM) are especially good for the heart, as is garlic (one clove a day).

Herbal infusions

Basil tones up the heart muscles. Camomile relaxes the mind and fenugreek lowers cholesterol. Amla (Indian gooseberry) in its natural form is high in vitamin C. You should take these herbs in infusions.

Exercises

As I mentioned in Chapter 6, yoga is the best form of exercise for the heart. There are several advantages, the main one being that these exercises are not strenuous and can be done even when the heart is repairing itself. On average the heart rate goes up by 10–15 per cent when doing yoga, compared to 100 per cent when doing aerobics. If required, and if the heart is able to take more strain, you can alter your breathing by retaining the air. In this case the heart is exercised thoroughly and the pulse rate goes up. After all, when doing the so-called aerobic exercises you are aiming to raise the heart rate by creating a demand for oxygen. By holding your breath during the various strenuous bodily movements, you create great demand for oxygen and so the heart rate goes up. The greatest advantage is that if there is any discomfort or pain in the chest, the breathing can be immediately altered and oxygen supply to the heart improved. During aerobic exercises, however, if there is any problem, it will be difficult to arrest the process as the heart will continue to beat vigorously for a while until the demand for oxygen is met.

Another great advantage is that yoga relieves stress, another desired effect for heart disease. The 'Shavasana' or dead man's posture (S4 on page 68) is clearly a highly meditative form of exercise. This is usually done at the end of a session of yoga.

For the heart I suggest the general daily exercises detailed on pages 64–73. These should be followed by Shavasana (S4), which can also be performed while still in the hospital after a heart attack, because it will slow down the heart rate and relax the body.

Brisk walking is a very good form of exercise for the heart. You must always do this in parks or open spaces where there is ample oxygen. **Tai Chi**, the Chinese form of exercise, is also very relaxing and puts the heart through sufficient strain to activate its muscles.

Medication

Conventional medicine has made great advances in the treatment of ischaemic heart disease. I think these should be used in preference to others available in traditional medicine. We know there are some side-effects, but the heart is such a vital organ that its role overshadows the role of all other organs.

Having said that, in India during the Mughal period, the court physicians were compelled to find cures for diseases that were similar to the ones that are prevalent in modern life. The Mughals led a decadent life indulging in food, alcohol, smoking and sex, and had many worries. They therefore suffered from ailments like high blood pressure, heart disease, diabetes, impotence, stress and arthritis. Their physicians were continuously searching for remedies for these ailments. That is why Unani medicine, the system that the Hakims in the Royal Court practised, had the best remedies for these conditions.

Using Avicenna's tips on cardiac medicine, Unani physicians compiled many remedies for the heart. They used silk cocoon, musk (from musk deer), minerals, herbs, and ashes of silver and gold to make special medicines. Some herbs such as Rauwolfia Serpentina, Valeriana and Digitalis went on to be researched and used in conventional medicine. Others remained untouched. Perhaps some pharmaceutical firms should look into these and study the efficacy of such herbs and minerals.

Heart failure (congestive heart failure)

Heart failure is an advanced complication of heart disease. The heart is an organ that pumps blood rhythmically. Any failure to do so causes circulatory problems. These may lead to accumulation of fluid in the legs or lungs, depending on where the failure takes place in the heart (left or right side). The weakness of the heart muscles caused by age, previous heart attacks or irregular rhythm of the heart are the main causes of heart failure. When the pump slows down there is flooding which puts an additional burden on the pump as the resistance increases.

Treatment

1

> **Strict Regimen Therapy** with a controlled diet, general massages, the general daily exercises detailed on pages 64–73, followed by Shavasana (S4), and stress management.

2

> **Conventional drugs** Ask your physician or cardiologist.

Prognosis

Heart failure is the ultimate warning that a person gets. If he or she does not change his or her lifestyle, then death is imminent. Fortunately modern techniques and drugs can keep the heart beating for a long time. One has to be prepared to take diuretics and digoxin-like drugs all the time to keep congestive heart failure under control.

Cardiac arrest

Cardiac arrest means simply that the heart has stopped. Death is imminent unless corrective action can be taken very quickly. Other people around may know what to do, but the worst case is when you are alone. Without help, the person whose heart stops beating properly and begins to feel faint has only about 10 seconds before losing consciousness. There is, however, hope.

The yoga exercise abdominal pump (E1), massages several internal organs, including the heart. Vigorous use of this exercise stands a good chance of getting the heart beating again, and has been used for this purpose for centuries. Another method has been recommended recently by researchers at Maryland University. They say that victims can help themselves by coughing repeatedly and very vigorously. A deep breath should be taken before each cough, and the cough must be deep and prolonged, as when producing sputum from deep inside the chest. A breath and a cough must be repeated about every two seconds without let up until help arrives, or until the heart is felt to be beating normally again. Deep breaths get oxygen into the lungs and the yoga exercise or coughing movements squeeze the heart and keep the blood circulating. The squeezing pressure on the heart also helps it to regain normal rhythm. This can give victims of cardiac arrest time to get to a phone and, between breaths, call for help.

Victims of heart disease would do well to practise the yoga exercise and the coughing so that they can be performed readily if the need arises. However, this is only a temporary solution. The sooner emergency medicine is applied the better it is. This includes CPR, fibrillator, and other emergency measures. Oxygen should be at hand.

Chapter

23

Prognosis

I have tried to show that integrated health, the gathering-together of all the best in medicine, leads to better, safer, more efficacious and cost-effective healthcare. It is so obvious, why hasn't anyone thought of it before?

Few could. To come to that conclusion requires experience in all the main modalities of medicine and healing worldwide. That is a tall order, and it wasn't until I came to write this book I realised that I had had the exceptional good fortune to come very near to that criterion myself, mostly by luck. I was able to observe folk medicine in India as I grew up, I studied and practised in Russia, and I worked for significant periods, mostly more than a year, in India, Thailand, Africa, Hong Kong (now China), the Middle East and Britain. During that time I came into contact with, and for the most part learned to practise, all the forms of treatment referred to in this book. Most importantly, I have been able to relate it to the budget overruns in the developed countries and see that only a return to the better and most effective traditional and conventional practices can save the profession. This has given me an extraordinary insight into health maintenance and healing. It enables me to declare unequivocally, what my Russian professor (Romashoff) instilled in me, that medicine has lost its way.

In all my experience in traditional medicine the overriding rule has always been, for thousands of years – stay as far as possible within the laws of nature. Throughout this book I have explained how medicine has become divorced from nature. It has upset the balances that exist in nature (through over-use of antibiotics, for example). It ignores the power of the physis, the role of the mind and the effect of the constitution and temperament in the individual's response to treatment.

Traditional and integrated medicine have always put health first, ensuring compliance with nature's law, the survival of the fittest. Their aim is to preserve quality of life up to as near the end of life as possible. This is compassionate and economical. Yet in modern societies it is common for 40 per cent of the 'health' budget to be spent on 5 per cent of the patients, ensuring the survival of the unfittest and leaving a miniscule amount to spend on prevention of illness and maintenance of health. Yet logic tells us it is better to invest in health than to spend on disease. Statistically, the nations who spend the most on healthcare are no healthier than those who spend the least. For every expensive scientific experiment that is successful there are four that fail. As a result 'health' services have become unsustainable 'disease' services and the only chance of survival of the various economies will be to integrate the best of all the treatments, and to start by making the best use of inexpensive Regimen Therapy, where the patient's participation is vital.

Conventional medicine should become integrated and focus on the three vital parameters, physical and emotional stress management (yoga), circulation (massage) and digestion (diet). The more simple the lifestyle, the healthier and the easier to treat people become. There needs to be a return to more physical treatment – hands on. Watch the animals: they touch, they lick, they scratch, they bite, roll over and play, even as adults, they chase for the sheer joy of exercise and the effect it has on their health, thus ensuring the survival of the fittest.

What will history say of us at the end of this century? Will they point to the twentieth century when we so overused antibiotics that we released super-deadly superbugs, bacteria and brought about a mutation in humans, causing a catastrophic vulnerabilty to viral and fungal infections? Will they say that we discarded the vast wealth of medical history and tradition in favour of a capricious excursion into science? Will they accuse us of departing from nature's law of the survival of the fittest by diverting a disproportionate amount of our assets towards the survival of the unfittest? Will there be a radical imbalance between the fitness of half the world who remain largely within the parameters of traditional medicine and the inherent weakness of the other half, resulting from their defiance of nature? Indeed, will our descendants look in the mirror and see the weaknesses that have evolved in their bodies and say 'Just look what our irresponsible ancestors did to us!'? Because that is the way we are going.

The way forward, the only way forward as I see it, is the introduction of integrated health ensuring the survival of the fittest, where most people come under that category, and where cures are carried out within nature's laws. Of course, such a radical step will not take place in this generation, whose ethic is to prolong life at any cost. It may not happen for several generations. But it will and must happen if the human race is to survive. It is a sobering thought that if drastic action is not taken and health services are allowed to become unsustainable, somebody is constantly going to have to choose between the middle-aged wastrel with self-imposed heart problems and a school full of children on an inadequate diet. The cost is about the same.

I believe that governments will have to undergo a total rethink on the objectives of their health services. They will have to divert far more of their resources to promote health, by teaching it as a compulsory and examinable subject in schools, by radical reform of the medical syllabus in colleges, by re-education of the general public and by the provision of health clinics in competition with the disease clinics they have today.

I don't know if they will make it by the next century but, there is no question, now is the time to start.

INDEX 1: Diseases and conditions

INDEX 2: General

A

acupuncture 128-9
   and backache 166
   and chronic fatigue 139
   and hypertension 147-8
adaptation (adaptogenic forces) 96-8
adolescence, and health 87-8
adrenalin 29, 183, 184, 185
adulthood, and health 88
age, effects on health 87-90
alcohol, effects on health 109-10, 219
Alexander Technique (posture therapy)
   165
allergies 48, 49, 130
   and headaches 171, 172, 173, 174
allopathic treatment 7 *see also*
   conventional medicine
antibiotics, long term problems 48,
   229-30
anxiety 95, 129, 130
auto-immune problems 130
Avicenna 16-18
Ayurvedic medicine 12, 18, 19-20, 140,
   166

B

back exercises 139
back surgery 167, 168
backache 112, 129, 130, 131, 158-69
   massage to help 79-80
   and stress 183
biorhythms 98-102
bloating (stomach) 47, 49, 109
blood pressure 108, 171, 172, 173 *see
   also* Index 1, hypertension
body
   biorhythms 99-100
   effects on mind 93-4
   smell 118
   effects of stress 185-7
bones 27
bowel function 109, 131
brain 27-8, 136-7
brain damage, and hypertension 144
brain haemorrhage 144
breath, smell from 109
breathing
   control of 26-7
   yoga 57-8
breathing rate, and health 108

C

caffeine, and sleep disorders 219
calcium supplements and vitamin D 140
carbohydrates 50
chemotherapy, for cancer 235, 236, 237
chewing food 47
children's ailments 87, 131
Chinese medicine 5-6, 12, 20-1, 100-1